Diy Homemade Healthy Living Projects

This Book Includes: Homemade Medical Face Mask And Homemade Hand Sanitizer. Everything You Need To Know About Hand Hygiene And Flu Protection For Adults And Kids

GABRIEL BLAKELY

Table of contents

Diy Homemade Medical Face Mask:

The Definitive Guide To Learn How To Make Easily Different Types Of Protective, Washable And Reusable Face Masks.

Step by Step Guide with Illustrations.

GABRIEL BLAKELY

Introduction

Ever since the pandemic has begun, you would have noticed that so many types of masks have been flying around. One thing is to be aware of your health status and how to protect it. It is another thing to know how to go about protecting yourself health-wise. You should know that not all the masks you see people wearing are what is right.

Most of these masks come in several specifications, which means none is adequate for all purposes. The most basic definition of a face mask is a mask that may or may not have a face shield but covers the nose and mouth. This does not guarantee you that it meets the required basic specification(s).

A dust mask may be beneficial while in a factory or an industrial setting. If you make use of this mask for medical purposes, it may not serve effectively. With a preference for tackling the pandemic virus, this book will walk you through the basic types of masks that fit in for this purpose. These masks are the N95 masks or Respirators, Surgical masks, and your homemade medical masks (made with cloth). These masks are still the most appropriate when it comes to minimizing the passage of the virus droplets into the mouth or the nose.

Before buying or before using a mask, you should consider some things. Face masks are not compulsory for everyone, though it can be used as a precautionary measure. Mostly, the use of Face masks should be employed by those who are sick and those working in the health sector. This is not to say that those are healthy should not use it, and it is just a matter of priority. People with infections like coughing, sneezing, or fever, in some cases, must make use of the masks to help curb spreading the Virus. Workers in the health sector too, are allowed to make use of the mask. This consists mostly of health workers that take care of people with respiratory diseases. It can also be those that are in close contact with people who have similar infections.

Considering these masks one by one, face masks or surgical masks are meant to prevent the user from spreading many droplets or sprays while coughing and sneezing. Making use of your homemade face mask apparently does the same thing as the Surgical Masks and the N95 masks.

Advantages and Disadvantages of Medical Masks

A clinical face mask has numerous potential points of interest. First of all, it very well may be a decent item to have in chilly climate. It helps in keeping a consistent temperature around your face. The breathed-out air flows in the chamber between your mouth and the mask and aides in keeping the face warm from outside boundaries of climate. masks additionally give a relief from the vast majority of the scents and smell one experience on an average every journey.

Face masks give security from external wellsprings of airborne contaminants. In urban areas where air contamination arrives at disturbing levels, these masks are successful in keeping out bigger residue and smoke particles. masks give a noteworthy favorable position against contracting respiratory maladies from beads and water fumes. A careful mask has different sides, which can be worn distinctively when you are ailing and would not have any desire to transmit that disease to other people, and when you are attempting to shield yourself from comparative difficulties.

These fill in as the primary apparatus in a medicinal services' proficient weapons store for security against microbes from infected patients and the social insurance setting. Face masks are practical and are effectively accessible from any comfort store or a drug store. For certain people, masks have become a concealment for the days when they are not in the temperament to make up and spruce up. In conclusion, it additionally gives a social separation when one is not feeling specific for meet and welcome. There are a few inconveniences to the utilization of a face mask as well.

In contrast to the respirators, face masks are expendable and lose adequacy subsequent to being worn for a couple of hours. The dampness in breathed out air diminishes the proficiency of the channels and prompts a higher molecule infiltration into the respiratory tract. Common face masks are additionally not viable in securing against littler measured infections and poisonous synthetic compounds. Face masks do not give adequate security against the fog and littler smoke particles. Careful face masks are likewise freely fitting in contrast with increasingly complex respirators. This leaves holes from where gases and other unsafe particles can enter.

In certain drug stores in urban regions, there are without a doubt numerous individual who purchase masks during this period. "It is essentially sold as dispensable masks. A few people purchase more than ten at once. At the point when they wear filthy, they discard it. Moderately, hardly any individuals utilize washed clinical masks. During this season's flu virus season, masks could be sure assume a job in antivirus, wearing a mask can fabricate a way between the human body and the outside world." The mask has a certain sifting impact broadcasting in real time entering the lungs, and it likewise has a specific obstruction capacity to the residue noticeable all around. In thickly populated regions, wearing a mask can hinder the attack of the infection. In the event that you have an abnormal body, wearing a mask is additionally liable for other people. Clinical staff at an emergency clinic in the urban region said that picking a dispensable mask is increasingly clean, cotton masks ought to be washed more. After each utilization, they should be cleaned once they return. Something else, the blocked residue and germs will likewise be sucked into the human body, which will not give security. Design masks sold in the city and in stores are not quite the same as clinical masks as far as material and thickness.

General masks can just assume the job of windproof and dustproof. Antivirus or clinical masks are progressively proficient. Simultaneously, clinical staff reminded that solid residents do not have to wear masks whenever, anyplace. They can build the body's opposition by opening more windows for ventilation in a shut space, eating a fair eating regimen, and practicing properly.

Chapter 1: Overview of Medical Masks

There is no evidence to prove the effectiveness of various measures, such as cleaning and disinfection of masks.

When purchasing and using medical surgical masks, they must be purchased from regular hospitals and pharmacies. At the same time, the outer packaging of the product must have the production batch number, date of production, and period of use. Information such as production license, product registration number, and detailed product use instructions must be found in the package.

- Always check if the packaging is undamaged before use, confirm the external packaging mark, production date, expiration date, and use it within the sterilization period.

- It should be ensured that the mask is covered with the bridge of the nose to the jaw after deployment to obtain the expected protective effect.

- Disposable medical surgical masks are prohibited from repeated usage.

- Use with caution to those who are allergic to nonwovens

- Medical-surgical masks should be handled in accordance with the requirements of hospitals and environmental protection departments after use.

Know How Masks Are Classified and Rated

N95 respirators, which have been reviewed, tested, and certified by the National Institute for Occupational Safety and Health (NIOSH), are typically the top-quality masks recommended for use in dental environments. N95 breathers filter at least 95% of the contaminants in the air and are forbidden for use in patients with or suspected of respiratory illness. Nevertheless, most dental procedures do not need N95 respirators, but maybe in medical therapy-diagnosis with adequate triages should be deferred until later on after patients have sufficiently stabilized from signs of respiratory diseases.

The American Society for Research and Materials (ASTM) sets standards of consistency and the components that are most commonly used in dental conditions of the face masks. The standards measure fluid resistance, performance in bacterial filtration, submicron particulate filtration performance, differential pressure and flame propagation. Each mask earns a ranking according to its level of safety, in compliance with the ASTM standards.

The ASTM evaluations are optional, but they are carried out by the top dental mask manufacturers. The ASTM F2100-11 specification includes a graphical representation of the mask output rating on the package.

Watch for packaging saying anything like "grade 2" may mean that the manufacturer did not personally check the masks.

Wear Your Mask Right-Side-Up and Right-Side-Out

A dental mask should have three layers: the outer layer is moisture resistant, the middle layer cleans, and the inner layer covers the nose. The textures inside and outside are not identical.

Dental practitioners wear their masks more inside than you might expect. If the masks are color-coded, the contrast between the inside and the outside is easy to see. Review the manufacturer's instructions for non-color-coded masks. Furthermore, manufacturers usually pack their masks face up with the outside.

Dental facial masks should suit the face's contours. Laps between your skin and a mask's edge can allow pollutants to enter. Your face mask must be focused on correctly.

Like a waterfall, the flaps on a face mask will face down.

A face mask may offer extra protection against sickness. The CDC advises, however, that you use masks only if you are advised by a doctor or if you have respiratory symptoms, like COVID-19, to prevent infection for others around you. There are no known threats beyond the expense of purchasing these products.

Don (Put On) Your Mask Correctly

Some people make the error as they place their masks over their heads first. But before you are securing your mask, make a small indentation or divot on your nose piece with your thumb. It helps better to place the mask on the bridge of the nose.

Open it a bit when you donate the mask (but not so much that the folds flicker). It makes the mask a perfect fit.

Then stretch the mask around the mouth and chin full. If you have a Stable Fit TM mask, change the bottom chin strap. This secures the exterior edges of the mask around the face and offers 360 degrees of security.

Often, practitioners with a broader face structure find like their masks are not adequately secure. They shorten the ear loops to compensate by making them into figure eight.

The concern is that the mask material is held up to the mouth and nose. Breath condensation travels inside the mask and allows the fibers of the mask material to swell in a process called wicking. In effect, this weakens the mask's ability to trap microbes. Using a Safe Fit mask is the best fit.

Take Off Your Mask Correctly

Much when there is a way to put on a face mask, there is a way to remove one. Incorrect removal of a tooth mask may lead to cross-contamination. Remember that the exterior surface of a face mask is coated with a film of aerosols, bacteria, blood bleeding and saliva. Place your fingertips under each ear loop above your ear lobes to make a face mask and pull straight back. Then remove the mask from the forehead and wash it. Should not contact the mask and use a mask even in the treatment room. Wash or using alcoholic hand rub shortly after the removal of the mask. Although masks seem to be promising, other prevention steps are also necessary. Make sure you always wash your hands — especially if you are with people who may be ill. Make sure that the yearly influenza shot prevents you and others from transmitting the infection.

Chapter 2: Steps On Cutting The Fabric

Before making a mask, clean your work area and hands

While creating a face mask, it is significant to have good hygiene. Clean your hands with soap and water for a minimum of 20 seconds to make sure that they are hygienic. Besides, you can also use bleach spray or bleach wipes to sterilize your work surface and tools.

- If you are creating masks to offer health care, think of wearing a mask whole, making them. In this way, you would not accidentally sneeze, cough, or breathe on the masks you are working on.

Choose a Tight-Woven, Heavy-Weight Fabric, like Cotton

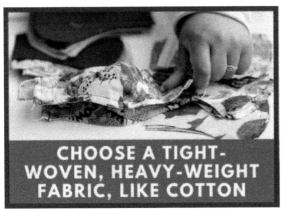

For better protection from microbes, you can pick a tight weave. If you like using a decorative fabric, you can. But you can also prefer using a heavy-weight pillowcase or T-shirt if you do not have any other material.

- If you are working on the purpose of donating the masks, you may get free supplies from any craft or a local fabric store near you. Many factories will provide you with the materials you require to make the masks FREE of charge.

Cut out the Fabric according to the Approved Pattern by CDC

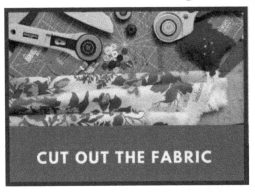

CDC (Central of Disease Control and Prevention) has given an average size of the face masks if you are making them at homes. After printing that actual size, you can check with the scale to make sure that you are proceeding in the right direction. For cutting out the fabric, use the sterilized scissors.

- Let me make it easy for you. Take a piece of fabric and cut out a rectangle with 20 cm (8 inches) tall and 18 cm (7 inches) wide. Reference the pattern given by the CDC as a guide while working. I know you can make this mask quite easily.

Copy the Pattern on the Fabric and Cut it

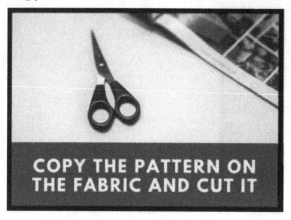

COPY THE PATTERN ON THE FABRIC AND CUT IT

Place the fabric on your workstation while putting the best side downwards. Put the sample pattern on the fabric. Take fabric chalk or a pencil and trace it around. After that, use sharp fabric scissors for cutting out the shape of a rectangle.

- Do not forget to keep the pattern adjacent as it will assist you in figuring out where you are going to fold the fabric while making the mask's body (central part).

For Ties, Cut Two Strips of Fabrics in Size 1.3 cm x 91.4 cm (0.5-inch x 36 inches)

The fabric ties play an important role in making the masks quickly because you do not need a lot of stuff for them. Also, you can easily alter your mask's fitting by loosening or tightening the ties. For cutting the tie, you can use the same fabric scissors.

- If you have a material having different colors or patterns, you can use different stuff for your ties.

- Variation: You may have seen some elastic straps. If you like those, you can use elastic as compared to the fabric. The elastic should be 0.95 cm (3/8 inch) or 0.64 cm (1/4 inch) wide. For each mask, you should have two strips.

Chapter 3: Step by Step Tutorial to Make Your Mask

Start Folding the Top 1.3 cm (0.5 inches) Edge of the Backside Over the Fabric Strap.

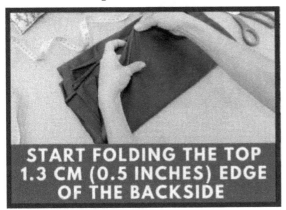

Put the material you are using for making the central part of the mask on your workplace with the 'right" side facing downwards. Place the fabric tie on the upper part of the rectangle. Do not forget to check that the strip of the fabric is at the center. Hence, there is an equal size on both sides of the mask. After that, fold the upper edge of the backside of the fabric over the fabric tie.

- You can line up the rough edge of the fabric with the fabric strip at the bottom to make sure that your straps stay in the right place.

Sew Along the Upper Part to Fix the Fabric Tie

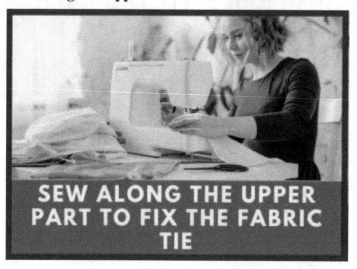

SEW ALONG THE UPPER PART TO FIX THE FABRIC TIE

Use a needle or sewing machine and sew to put some straight stitches around the rough edge of the fabric. Do all the way around from one end of the fabric to the other. Just leaves the sides open; hence you can add a wire later.

- This straight stitch can hold the fabric strap in place and leave a small space at the upper part of the mask.

- Variation: If you are using elastic, you need to fold the upper part of the backside of fabric down and sew like a tunnel around the mask's top. After that, enclose a stripped twisty tie or a metal floral wire in the center of the shaft. The next step is to use a straight stitch for attaching one end of an elastic part at the edge of the tunnel. At last, sew some consecutive stitches for connecting one end of the other flexible piece on the other side of the tunnel.

Add Metal Floral Wire in the Pocket at the Upper Part of the Mask

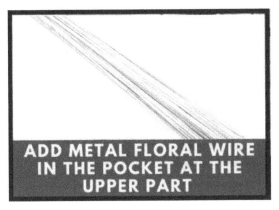

Take the floral wire and cut about 14 cm (5.5 inches). In the tunnel which you just made now, slide the metal wire down the top strap. For pushing the wire in place at the upper portion of the mask, use your fingers. This wire will permit the wearer to adjust the cover around the nose. If there is no metallic wire, you can also use a twisty tie. Do not forget to strip off the paper. It will come off while washing if you do not.

To Create Pleats, Make Small Folds (maximum 3) at the Center of the Mask

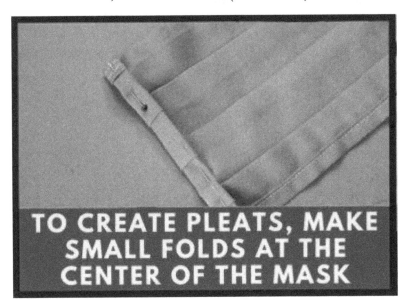

The pleats assist in setting the mask according to the face of the wearer. You should make the first fold about 1.3 cm (0.5 inches) below the top of the

cover. After that, make another 1.3 cm (0.5 inches) fold and make sure that pleat in place with the help of a pin. Keep doing the same process for making a total of three pleats. At the bottom, you can leave about 2.5 cm (1 inch) so that it will be easy to attach the other tie.

- Make use of a mask pattern as your guide for creating the pleats so that everything can go the right way.

To Secure the Wire and Pleats, Stitch up the Sides

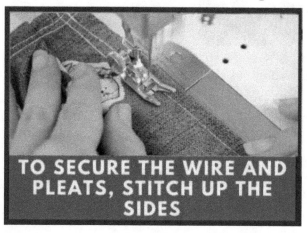

After folding all the three pleats, fold the edges of the fabric from the front side about 0.64 cm (0.25 inch) towards the back. After that, start sewing the straight stitches on every side to make the side seams. It will not only make your pleats secure but also prevent the wire on the area of the nose from falling out.

- Remember to use the pattern as a reference.

Start Folding the Bottom 1.3 cm (0.5 inches) over the Second Strip of Fabric

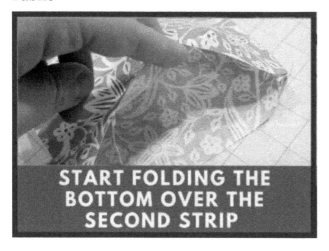

Put the second strip of fabric over the bottom of the mask. Always make sure that the strip is in the center; hence there are equal amounts of straps on both sides of the cover. After that, fold the lower edge of the mask's backside over the strip of fabric. Line up the rough edge with the upper side of the strip. Then, secure the mask around the bottom strap through sewing stitches along the jagged line.

- It is precisely the same as the first step for creating the mask.

- Variation: Instead of fabric strips, if you are using the elastic, fold the bottom 1.3 cm (0.5 inches) of the backside of the mask and sew around the rough edge utilizing a straight stitch for making another tunnel. Beginning from the right side, insert the free elastic end you linked at the top of the mask into the tunnel and use the straight stitches for sewing it in place. After that, do the same on the left side. It will make ear loop on both sides of the mask.

Sew the Topstitch Around the Perimeter of the Mask Two Times to Secure it

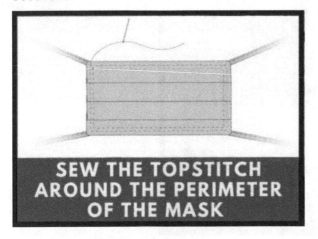

Use a hand sewing needle or sewing machine and thread to complete all the topstitch. It will decrease the chance of your mask coming apart or fraying.

If you are in a hurry, you can skip the topstitch. But if you add a topstitch, your mask will hold up better in the wash.

Wash the Mask Before Wearing it

If your mask is dirty, your cover cannot protect you from the microbes. Wash it in detergent for sanitizing it. After that, dry it in the dryer for the best results. You can air-dry your mask if necessary. But heat can kill more microorganisms. Hence it is the best thing to use a dryer.

Sanitize the mask by boiling it for 10 minutes if you do not have a washing machine. After that, place it on a clean surface to dry.

Chapter 4: Analyzing and Comparing Homemade Materials and Masks

Comparison of Homemade Materials

While a few pundits contend that utilizing natively constructed material for assurance against microorganisms is not viable, accessible research material reports in any case. An examination led at Cambridge University tried the viability of custom-made masks, as an option in contrast to industrially accessible masks (Davies et al. 2013). To gauge the adequacy of the masks, microscopic organisms estimated between 0.93-1.25 microns were taken shots at various family unit materials. Twenty-one volunteers enrolled for the exploration and microorganisms were confined from their hack to confirm the dis-mask. It was dis-masked that in spite of the fact that the careful masks were progressively compelling in blocking transmission, masks produced using vacuum cleaner sacks, dish towels and a cotton mix texture were effective in blocking microorganism at 95%, 83% and 74% separately.

Analyzing of Homemade Materials and Masks

The economically accessible careful mask was compelling in blocking 97% of particles. The examination further tried whether particles, five-times littler than the current respiratory infection causing devastation all around, can be adequately sifted through. The respiratory infection segregated from the ongoing episode is estimated at around 0.1 microns. A bacteriophage estimating 0.02 microns, at any rate multiple times littler was taken shots at the masks. The investigation reasoned that the various materials tried were by and large, 7% less powerful separating this size against the bigger microorganisms utilized already. The careful mask was 89% powerful, while family things, for example, vacuum cleaner sacks, dish towels and cotton mix texture were 86%, 73% and 70% viable separately (Davies et al. 2013). To additionally test an alternate system for adequacy, the analysts had a go at utilizing a twofold layer to evaluate the separating quality of natively constructed masks.

A similar infection measured particles were taken shots at the masks. While just a peripheral 1% sifting viability expanded for pillowcase and cotton mix, the drying towel masks indicated a stunning 14% expansion in separating capacity. 97% of particles separated by twofold layered dish towels were at standard with the viability of a careful mask. In any case, it was presumed that albeit incredible at separating off little estimated microorganisms. The vacuum cleaner pack and dish towels are not an incredible decision for managing it-yourself face masks, because of the way that these materials are not breathable enough. The scientists in the examination tried the drop in pressure with each sort of texture utilized, to give a decent comprehension of the solace related during relaxing. The outcomes indicated that while twofold layered dish towels and vacuum cleaner packs were 128% and 104% harder to take in when contrasted with a careful face mask, a cotton mix twofold layered was 3% simpler to take in against a similar control.

Another little investigation utilized paper towels as the primary material for making a hand-crafted mask. In spite of the fact that it is the broadly accessible material utilized in every single hand-crafted item, the dis-masks indicated that a paper towel was just 33% compelling in sifting particles of 0.3 microns in size (Robertson 2020). This reason paper towels are not so viable in sifting through infections and different microorganisms.

Chapter 5: Other Protective Measures against Microorganisms

While face masks play an important protective role, some other measures also benefit widely in protecting against bacterial infections.

Hygiene

Personal hygiene plays an integral role in protecting ourselves and others from illness. This includes washing hands with a potent antibacterial soap or a sanitizer, disposing of germ-laden tissue papers and sanitary items in closed dustbins and covering your mouth while sneezing or coughing. Bathing is also important in warding off germs, cleaning oneself at least every day and using deodorants to stop body smells play a key role in maintaining personal hygiene. Body smells are caused by sweating, metabolism waste products excreted onto our skins, unwashed clothes and undergarments. Most infections, such as common cold and food poisoning occur when unwashed hands are used for eating or preparing the food. Hands and wrists should be cleaned using an alcohol-based soap for at least 20 seconds. Fingernails should be kept short and brushing can help in dislodging dirt stuck in the nails. You should always be dried after washing with a paper towel or a dryer. Women require special hygiene attention due to different sanitary conditions. During menstruation, care must be taken in washing hands after handling tampons or sanitary pads. Regularly washing the genital areas can protect against infections of the genitalia. Urinating after sexual intercourse helps in flushing out bacteria and avoiding conditions like cystitis. Men who have not gone circumcision have a build-up of secretions known as smegma. Pulling the skin back and cleaning these secretions is important in preventing Urinary Tract Infections. Good dental hygiene is vital for protection from diseases of gums and teeth. Brushing teeth properly and flossing regularly helps against bad breath and infections. Using approved mouthwashes and chewing gums also aid but having regular checkups with a dentist is most important. While travelling overseas to places where sanitary conditions are not up to the mark, additional care must be taken to ensure that water being used is safe for consumption. Avoid using tap water for drinking and cleaning fruits or vegetable purposes. If bottled water is not available, boil the available water for at least a minute before using it. Boiling the water kills most bacteria and pathogens.

Immunization

Vaccination plays a key role in training the immune system for identification and combating of pathogens such as viruses or bacteria. Introducing some molecule from the pathogen triggers an immune response from the body. These introduced molecules, known as antigens, after entering the body elicit a response from body's immune cells to develop antibodies. Whenever the bacteria virus reappears, the body immediately recognizes and aggressively attacks the pathogen with a speed greater than the earlier mounted response. This curtails the pathogen and prevents it from causing any serious illness. Immunization protects individuals from serious illnesses such as polio, pneumonia, diphtheria, tetanus, measles, mumps and pertussis to name a few. In immunocompromised and unvaccinated children, the severity of such infections can lead to serious complications, even death in some cases. Vaccines are developed after much deliberation and review by scientists, researchers and healthcare professionals. Therefore, they are very safe and effective in preventing serious diseases. Some local side effects such as pain, tenderness and rash at the site of infection might occur but this is a much lower cost when compared to pain and discomfort associated with the disease which is being prevented. Vaccination has led to a great reduction and even elimination of certain infections such as smallpox and polio. Polio still remains active in two countries. Immunization is much more cost-effective when compared to the treatment of the disease. Immunized individuals in a community lead to a lower risk of development of an epidemic or a pandemic.

Nutrition

Nutrition and diet play a key role in the development and action of the immune system against infectious diseases. The nutritional status of a body is intricately linked to the immune response a body will be able to mount. Over nutrition and malnutrition, both can leave a person susceptible to the implications and complications of diseases. Malnutrition results from inadequacy in protein, caloric and micro-nutritional intake. This disturbs the blood chemistry, lean muscle proportion and functioning of various organs. Malnutrition has been linked to increased morbidity and mortality. Foods rich in minerals and vitamins such as fruits and vegetables prove beneficial during an infection. The antioxidant ability of Vitamin C, which is abundantly found in citric fruits, aids the body's immune system against free radical formation as a result of pathogenesis. Keeping the body hydrated counters the effects of fever and infection. Infections can also be transmitted through foodborne pathogens. These result from improper preparation and storage of food. The following precautions can help in avoiding microbial infiltration into our food cycles. Rinsing poultry, fruits, vegetables, fish and meat products underwater before cooking can help wipe off any microbes or other chemicals such as insecticides and pesticides. Always properly wash your hands with a potent antiseptic soap and water before handling food, especially the meat products. Cook meat products under sufficient heat to get rid of any pathogen. Undercooked food is a leading cause of gastrointestinal infections.

Antibiotics

Antibiotics have become a very common medication prescribed to fight against bacteria. Proper use of antibiotics can play a lifesaving role against infections. Antibiotics act by either stopping the reproduction of bacteria or by destroying them completely. Antibiotics come in all preparations, such as over the counter oral drugs, creams, ointments and also in intravenous formulations. However, there is a growing concern with the overuse of antibiotics, which many doctors believe is leading to the development of mutations and resistance. This has led to many bacteria becoming strong enough to evade the action of antibiotics. Some antibiotics are prescribed against aerobic bacteria, while others against anaerobic bacteria. Antibiotics are also often prescribed prophylactically before surgical procedures. There are a few side effects associated with the use of antibiotics which include diarrhea, nausea, vomiting, rash and upset stomach. Much less commonly, the formation of kidney stones, abnormal blood clotting, sensitivity to sunlight, blood disorders and deafness can occur with some particular antibiotics. However, the side effects when weighed against the benefits of antibiotics are mostly of insignificant value.

Analyzing and Comparing Homemade Material and Masks While some critics argue that using homemade material for protection against microorganisms is not effective, available research material reports otherwise. A study conducted at Cambridge University tested the efficacy of homemade masks, as an alternative to commercially available masks (Davies et al. 2013). To measure the effectiveness of the masks, bacteria sized between 0.93-1.25 microns were shot at different household materials. Twenty-one volunteers enlisted for the research and microorganisms were isolated from their cough to verify the findings. It was found that although the surgical masks were more effective in blocking transmission, masks made from vacuum cleaner bags, dish towels and a cotton blend fabric were successful in blocking microorganism at 95%, 83% and 74% respectively. The commercially available surgical mask was effective in blocking 97% of particles. The study further tested whether particles, five-times smaller than the current respiratory virus causing havoc globally, can be sufficiently filtered out. The respiratory virus isolated from the recent outbreak is measured at around 0.1 microns. A bacteriophage measuring 0.02 microns, at least 5 times smaller was shot at the masks. The study concluded that the different materials tested were on average, 7% less effective filtering this size against the larger bacteria used previously. The surgical mask was 89% effective, whereas household items such as vacuum cleaner bags, dish towels and cotton blend fabric were 86%, 73% and 70% effective respectively (Davies et al. 2013). To further test a different strategy for effectiveness, the researchers tried using a double layer to assess the filtering strength of homemade masks. The same virus sized particles were shot at the masks. While only a marginal 1% filtering effectiveness increased for pillowcase and cotton blend, the dish towel masks showed a staggering 14% increase in filtering ability. 97% of particles filtered by double-layered dish towels were at par with the effectiveness of a surgical mask. However, it was concluded that although great at filtering off small-sized microorganisms. The vacuum cleaner bag and dish towels are not a great choice for making do-it-yourself face masks, due to the fact that these materials are not breathable enough. The researchers in the study tested the drop in pressure with each type of fabric used, to give a good understanding of the comfort associated during breathing. The results showed that while double layered dish towels and vacuum cleaner bags were 128% and 104% harder to breathe in when compared to a surgical face mask, a cotton blend double-layered was 3% easier to breathe in against the same control. Another small study used paper towels as the main material for making a homemade mask. Although it is the widely available material used in all homemade products, the findings showed that a paper towel was only 33% effective in filtering particles of 0.3 microns in size (Robertson 2020). This concludes that paper towels are not that effective in filtering out viruses and other microorganisms.

Science Behind Hand Sanitizers

The two active ingredients in the hand sanitizer: 60% ethanol and 70% isopropanol share some genetic language with certain disease-causing viruses, which then result in their deactivation. Alcohol is composed of carbon, hydrogen, and oxygen. The common types of alcohol are easily soluble in water, which are ethanol (mainly used in alcoholic drinks), isopropanol (mainly found in disinfectants), and propanol. The exact process through which alcohol kills germs is by destroying its metabolism or by splitting the microbe's cells.

You can find hand sanitizers with varying percentages of alcohol content, from 30% to 95%. A solution with 30% alcohol content will definitely manage to kill certain microbes, but it will not be as effective as a solution with 70% or 90% alcohol content. The effectiveness increases with strength. That is why it is recommended to use a sanitizer with a minimum 60% alcohol content. However, with a higher concentration of 95%, the solution might get saturated.

Bacteria species such as Escherichia coli, Serratia marcescens, and Staphylococcus saprophyticus are easily affected by ethanol. Another benefit of using a hand sanitizer on a regular basis is the inability of the harmful bacteria and viruses to develop a resistance power against the alcohol solution irrespective of the long duration of exposure. This is why you can keep on using hand sanitizers and achieve the same results. In fact, a hand sanitizer with a higher ethanol percentage is said to be more effective than washing your hands. However, hand sanitizers are not 100% effective in killing all kinds of bacteria, certain heavy metals, and some pesticides. Therefore, do not overestimate its use and practice other hygienic routines as well. Speaking of the expiration dates of these hand sanitizers, there is not really a specific expiration time. The labels only show an expiration date because these are under the regulation of the FDA. However, your sanitizer solution might weaken over time. This is because alcohol can evaporate easily due to its low boiling point. Even if ethanol has a longer shelf life, it is recommended to store it an air-tight container to conserve its strength. If you are using a bottle, try to avoid opening and closing it frequently to protect it from evaporating.

Chapter 6: How to Wear The Mask Correctly

Before you wear your homemade mask, follow the tips below:

1. Wash the mask before you use it.

2. Wash your hands before putting on a mask

3. Do not reuse a mask without first washing it

4. Once the mask becomes humid or damp, switch to a different mask and wash the used one.

When removing a mask:

1. Remove the mask using the strings or the band behind. Do not touch the front of the mask or any surface of the face mask.

2. If removing a string mask, first untie the string below before you untie the one above.

3. After you take off a mask, wash your hands under running water and soap for at least forty seconds. Alternatively, use a hand sanitizer with at least 60 percent alcohol content.

4. Drop used masks in a soap solution immediately you take it off. Wash the mask thoroughly before you use it again.

Other tips

5. Use a face mask only when outside your home. Do not use the mask at home or in the car. Only when in public places like the supermarket where it may be hard to practice social distancing.

6. Do not take off your mask until you get home, or you get to a place where you can wash your hands as well as practice social distancing.

7. Advisable to remove the paper towel inserts before you soak your face mask. This is for the face masks that are not sewn.

8. Do not go to public places if you have any symptoms like fever, cough, or stuffy nose.

9. Lastly, do not go out if you have no urgent business outside.

Mask Wearing Rules and Guidelines for Care

Wearing a medical mask is a preventative measure for protecting yourself against diseases, viruses, germs, and bacteria. However, using a mask as your only protective means is not enough. Besides wearing a mask, you must follow hand hygiene rules and other requirements for the prevention and control of the contagion.

When you are using medical masks, it is important to follow the proper usage guidelines and disposal rules in order to ensure their utmost efficiency and avoid an increased risk of virus transmission. Based on experiences from practical medical practice, the following recommendations have been developed for proper use of medical masks:

1) Put your mask on carefully, so that it covers your mouth and nose, and tightly secure it, minimizing the gaps between the face and the mask.

2) Avoid touching the mask while you are wearing it.

3) Take the mask off without touching the front part of it, using elastic bands at the back.

4) After taking the mask off, sanitize your hands or wash them with soap.

5) As soon as the mask becomes wet, replace it with a new one – clean and dry. (This applies to reusable masks only!)

6) Do not reuse disposable masks.

7) Immediately after use, throw the masks away into a waste container.

It is important to keep in mind that taking the following precautions may be more important for self-protection than the mask-wearing.

For healthy people:

Keep your distance when talking to a person with flu-like symptoms, and:

- Avoid or reduce the time spent in crowded areas.

- Try not to touch your mouth and nose.
- Follow the hand hygiene rules — wash your hands daily with soap and water or use sanitizer, particularly if you touch your mouth and nose, or potentially dangerous surfaces.
- Reduce time of close contact with people who may be ill.
- Increase the inflow of fresh air into areas of your home.

For people with flu-like symptoms:

- Try to keep your distance from healthy people.
- If you do not feel well, stay at home and follow your doctor's recommendations.
- Close your mouth and nose when coughing and sneezing with a handkerchief, or other materials suitable for this purpose, to stop the spreading from the respiratory tract. Dispose of this material immediately after use or wash it. Wash your hands immediately after contact with respiratory secretions!
- Ventilate the patient's room as often as possible.

When wearing masks, it is extremely important to use and dispose of them properly. This will increase their efficiency and avoid an increased risk of disease transmission.

Some viral infections can transmit through a mucous membrane of eyes; therefore, wearing protective eye masks increases the level of your protection as well.

Chapter 7: How to Make an Effective Face Mask?

Masks

The public is recommended to not purchase surgical masks or N95 respirators (or any other respirator for that matter) since they are required by healthcare professionals, who cannot follow social distancing protocols and are completely exposed to the virus.

But in the absence of masks, what can one do? Well, they can make use of homemade masks.

The most important point to remember is that social distancing should be your primary priority. Personal hygiene, like effective handwashing, is vital. Masks are only meant to protect you during an emergency situation, not to support outdoor activities that are not necessary under the given circumstances.

One of the misconceptions people have about homemade masks is the complexity involved in making them. Mention the phrase "homemade masks" and people think of sewing machines and pondering what trouser or dress they have to sacrifice in order to make the masks.

The tips given help you prepare masks that require limited knowledge of sewing. This means that you will not have to worry about trying to follow a complex process.

However, if you do know how to sew, then I am going to provide some instructions for you as well.

No Sewing Method

Let us start with the materials that you will require for this method. You need only three items:

- I would prefer if you got a bandana. However, you can cut out a square cloth from any material that you have, especially old shirts. Ideally, you are looking for a cloth that is 20 inches by 20 inches.

- Ties or rubber bands.

- Coffee filter

But some of you might be wondering what you can do when you do not have coffee filters. Well, you use the paper towel method.

Enjoying this book?

Please leave a review because we would love to hear your feedback, opinions and advice to create better products and services for you! Thank you for your support. You are greatly appreciated!"

The paper towel method

The beautiful thing about this method is that you can use it for not just making masks, but anytime you would like to filter some of your coffee. Here is how you do it:

Step 1

Take a square paper towel. Bring two corners of the paper towel together such that you now have a triangle.

You can either use coffee filters or make filters of your own.

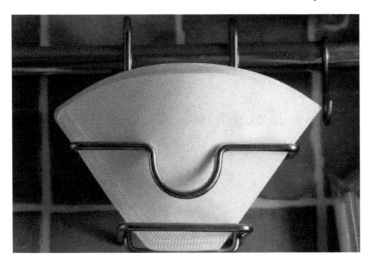

Step 2

In the triangle that you just formed; one side will be longer than the remaining two. Place the triangle in such a way that the longest side becomes the bottom of the triangle.

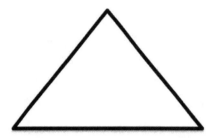

You will roughly get a triangular shape. Make sure the longest side is at the bottom.

Step 3

You now have one angle pointed up, with two angles pointed to the sides.

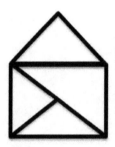

Bring the left angle to the right side of the triangle and the right angle to the left side. When you bring the two angles together, make sure that the top of those two angles are on the same level.

This is a rough representation of what the paper towel should look like.

Step 4

At this point, you will notice that the top angle is still pointing up. This angle will have multiple layers of the paper towel. Take one layer and then fold it towards you. Fold the remaining layers away from you.

And that is it. You have made your very own coffee filter, soon to be a mask filter.

Making the Mask

Time to make the mask itself. For this, follow the steps below.

<u>Step 1</u>

Lay the cloth or bandana out in front of you and fold it lengthwise. Unfold the bandana and note the crease running through the middle.

Step 2

Place the coffee filter—or your makeshift filter—on the crease. Align the filter as close to the center as possible. Once you have found the right alignment, you have three sections on the cloth. The middle section is occupied by the filter. You will have an empty space on top, which is the top section of the cloth. Then you have an empty space at the bottom of the cloth, which is the bottom section. All you have to do now is fold the top section of the cloth or bandana over the filter. Next, fold the bottom section of the cloth over the top.

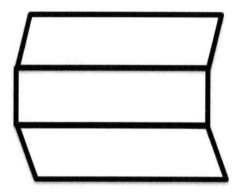

The center section of the cloth or bandana will have your filter. Once you place the filter, fold the cloth according to the instructions in Step 2. You should have a single strip of cloth.

Step 3

Place two rubber bands around the folded cloth or bandana. There should be around 6 inches of space between the rubber bands, and they should be arranged with equal space remaining on the ends of the cloth or bandana.

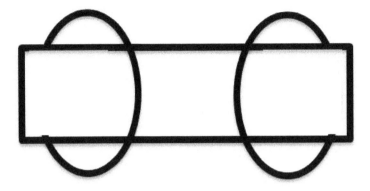

Bring the elastic materials on either side of the fabric.

Step 4

Fold the ends of the cloth or bandana over the rubber bands and towards the middle. If the two ends of the cloth do not meet in the middle, you do not have to worry about that fact. The most important aspect of the makeshift mask is that it should fit comfortably on your face.

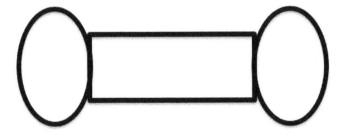

Sometimes, you might not be able to get the two ends of the fabric right in the center when you fold them. Adjust the placement of the elastic materials to get the correct alignment.

Step 5

Put on the mask. If it fits snugly on your face, then you have created a good mask. Make any adjustments necessary to create the right fit.

TIPS

If you prefer, you can create a bunch of masks in advance. Once you do, you can follow the below tips.

- Once you make new masks, place them in a container. Arrange them in such a way that it is easy for you to take them out, which will prove useful when you have to step out in a hurry.

- Keep separate containers for used masks, one for each member of the house. This way, you can place your used mask inside a container meant for you, minimizing further exposure to germs or particles. A simple trick to make sure that people do not accidentally use another person's mask is to use a marker and draw a small mark on the cloth. You can use a different colored marker for a different cloth.

- What happens when you wash the cloth mask and are drying them? Take out a new mask, which then becomes yours. When the older mask is dry, transfer it to a container meant for you. When you wash the new mask, then you can take out the older one that is now in your container. Perform this tip for each member in the house.

- Make sure that you do not transfer a damp cloth or bandana to your container. Allow them to dry completely before placing them anywhere.

- You can even label the containers to help others know where they should go if they would like a mask.

Sewing Method

Let us look at the materials required for the job.

- A cotton cloth or fabric that is tightly woven

- Rubber bands or other elastic materials (such as hair ties, cloth strips, or strings)

- A sewing machine (or you can use a needle and thread—the task is not going to be to0 daunting or complex)

- Scissors

Once you have the necessary materials, simply follow the below steps.

<u>Step 1</u>

Cut all your fabrics into the same dimensions, which should be 10 inches by 6 inches. Align the fabrics on top of each other.

<u>Step 2</u>

Focus on the longer sides. Fold about a quarter of an inch of the length inwards. Sew them in using the machine or the needle and thread. You do not have to make a complex stitch; a simple hem will suffice. Make sure you follow this step for both of the longer sides of your cloth.

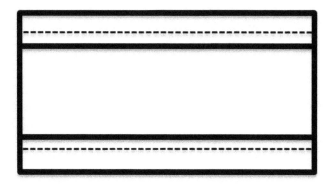

You will have folded the longer sections and stitched them.

<u>Step 3</u>

Next, fold the shorter sides inward; about a half-inch fold will do. Stitch these sides as well.

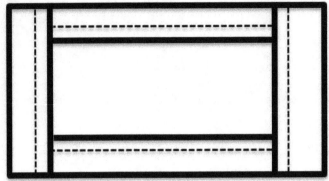

Make sure that when you are stitching the shorter sides in, you leave an opening in the middle.

Once you have completed your stitch, there should be a hollow running down the shorter side.

The stitches made on the sides should be close to the innermost edge, leaving a hollow between the stitch and the outer edge.

Step 4

Run the elastic material that you have into the hollow. It would be ideal if you have a material that is at least 6 inches long.

Step 5

Once you have run the elastic band or material through the hollow, create a knot to secure it. If you have rubber bands, then you have to cut them, run them through the hollow and then secure them.

Step 6

Start tugging at the elastic material gently in order to slowly slide the knot into the hollow. You do not have to slide the knot all the way to the middle of the hollow. The main purpose is to hide the knot.

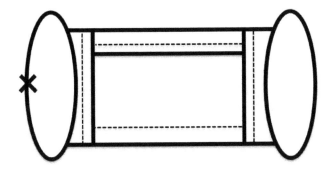

After you run the elastic materials through the hollows, secure them with a knot. Slowly move the elastic materials until the knots disappear into the hollow portion.

Step 7

Wear the mask and see if it fits properly on your face. If it does not, do not try to remove the knot and tie it again, since it could weaken the strength of the material. Rather, cut it and remove it entirely in order to use a new elastic material. You only have to do this process the first time, since you will know just how long the material should be in order to give you a comfortable fit. Once you know the length, you can replicate it on other elastic bands.

And that is all there is to it. You have made your very own face mask.

TIPS

- Make sure that the elastic material that you use has great tensile strength. In other words, it should not snap easily when stretched. I would recommend getting an elastic band that is at least ⅛ inch thick. That should give the band sufficient strength to hold your mask together.

- You can be creative with the face mask itself, should you wish to. Use different colored fabrics with unique designs to get a colorful output. I do understand that talking about unique face masks might seem odd at the moment, but the one thing that we should not fall into is a state of gloom. At a time such as this, it is important that we keep our spirits up, even if it means trying to make a face mask look good.

- If the masks become damp even though you did not wash them, then consider changing the mask entirely.

- Create multiple masks and use the suggestions of No Sewing Method to create separate containers for each person living in your house. Take your time to get the stitches right so that you have a secure mask for you to use. In many cases, you will not be able to re-stitch the materials. By making proper stitches, I am not talking about technique. Rather, if your stitches are wrong, then you might have a mask that tears easily.

Chapter 8: Why We Need to Avoid Touching Our Face?

Viruses become diseases when they get into your body from your hands. You may become infected if you touch infected surfaces and then touch your eyes, nose, or mouth.

The problem is that you mostly do not notice when you touch your face. We often automatically support our face in the palm of our hand, rub an itchy eye, or touch our lips.

The following tips will help you touch your face less often:

Find out how you mostly touch your face and find an alternative.

Use scented soap to notice when your hands come close to your face.

Ask others to let you know when you touch your face.

Wash your hands when it is necessary to touch your face.

Use a clean handkerchief to avoid contact with your skin if you cannot wash your hands.

How to Take Care of an Infected Person and Protect Yourself during a Pandemic Outbreak

If someone in your family gets flu, there is a high chance that other people in the family will be infected if you do not take precautions. At the same time, you will also be worried and want to take care of the

sick person. By following these tips, you will reduce the risk to yourself and the rest of the family and ensure that you stay healthy enough to take care of the sick person.

Make sure that the sick person stays in a room because s/he will exhale viruses, cough, and touch surfaces. If s/he stays in a room, the viruses cannot spread around the house.

Clean surfaces on which there could be viruses. A large number of viruses will accumulate near the forehead of the sick person (e.g., handkerchiefs, as well as on upholstery, your clothes, and towels). Surfaces that are touched are also infected (e.g., toys, glasses, door handles).

Always have enough handkerchiefs and trash cans to dispose of. This means that every family member can use and dispose of clean handkerchiefs without

spreading viruses to others. If you do not have enough rubbish bins, you can place plastic bags next to the sick person's bed. These bags can then be thrown directly into the dung bucket.

Then wash your hands.

Try to stay 1m away from the family member with the flu. Studies have shown that viruses cover a distance of 1m in the air when they are exhaled. If you keep as much distance as possible, you will reduce the number of viruses you come into contact with.

Try to limit the time you spend in the same room with the sick person. The likelihood of getting infected is increased if you spend too much time in rooms with a high number of viruses.

How to Stay Positive during a Pandemic

When there is a virus epidemic, everyone talks about it, and they are bound to worry.

All your favorite activities are canceled, and your favorite places are closed. How should you handle this situation? Here are a few tips:

1. Stay active

It is important to do 30 minutes of physical activity, both for your physical and mental health. You could take a walk, do some stretching or yoga, play active video games, or dance. Whatever activity you choose, the important thing is to get active.

Do something you enjoy doing or try

something new. Set a new goal, such as doing 10 push-ups, reaching for your toes without bending your knees, or learning a new dance number. Share your goal with others and post photos or updates of your progress so others can encourage you.

2. Have fun

Do things that make you feel good. You could go to play outside or read a book inside. Be creative and make a craft item.

Draw, write or make music. These are all things that will help you feel better and relax. You might even find fun things online that would allow you to continue doing the activities that you enjoy. For example, you could check online for dance companies that offer free live dance lessons online.

3. Keep your routine

Even if you cannot go anywhere because of job and school closings and the cancellation of certain activities, it is important to keep up some semblance of a routine. On weekdays, wear clothes that you would usually wear during the day.

Reserve pajamas for the weekend. Establish a schedule each day, incorporating physical activity, learning, fun, contacting friends and family, and time of tranquility. It is also vital to sleep well, exercise, and eat healthy foods every day.

4. Get your brain working

For the kids, closing schools does not mean you have to stop learning. Do any kind of learning activity every weekday. Your teachers may send you homework that you can do, or you can find learning activities.

5. Try to stay calm

It is entirely understandable to be worried about a pandemic or to be sad because of the repercussions a virus spread can have on your life. If you think you are too stressed and may need help, you can talk to your friends, family or another trusted adult.

6. Stay in touch

Even if we are all asked to stay away from each other, that does not mean that you cannot communicate with your friends. You need to keep in touch with these people. Reach your loved ones by utilizing technology. Chat them via any social network of your choice. Anything that works for you and your family can be used. You could even teach one of your grandparents to use this means of communication so that they can stay in touch!

7. Help around

Knowing your family has a plan can help you feel more secure. Talk to your loved ones about the plans they have in place to stay as safe as possible. Ask if there is anything you can do to help them. They could give you some chores at home, like making sure everything is well cleaned.

8. Stay on top of the facts

It may be helpful to know more about the pandemic, how to protect yourself from it, the symptoms of the disease, and what to do if you feel sick. There is a great deal of information about a pandemic. Still, it is essential to make sure that you inquire from reliable sources.

However, do not spend too much time watching, reading, or listening to the news. It can become depressing to hear too much about a pandemic.

Chapter 9: Why We Should Know The Importance Of Face Mask

Importance of face mask

The primary purpose of a face mask is to prevent the fluid from the mouth or nose of an infected individual (gross, I know). You can be prevented from being sick by taking it, because you are in direct contact with someone who is infected, will keep you from transmitting the illness to anyone else. The biggest advantage of wearing a mask is that it lets you avoid sickness and therefore lets you stay functioning. In particular, it avoids the growth that could reduce quality and length of life, of diseases that could damage your airways.

Use a mask you can avoid signs of lung illness from inhaling harmful conditions (such as cough, wheezing, breathability, chest tightness or trouble breathing).

An additional 12,000 deaths were reported in 2009/10 and 12,000 deaths were reported in 2010/11 from long-term respiratory problems.

Tight-fitting N95 respirator masks block large contaminants from accessing your mouth and provide you with much more effective protection against airborne disease. These two masks can help you protect against an infection with the virus.

Types of masks (REUSUABLE)

1.   Surgical mask

Over wearing is meant to be used by health practitioners during service and during necessity to absorb blood droplets and aerosols from the mouth and nose of the wearer, commonly known as an operating mask, surgical mask or simply as a face mask. These do not shield wearers from airborne bacteria and virus particle inhalation, and they are less effective than breathers such as N95 or FFP masks which, by their design, form and tight seal provide better protection.

2. N-95 respirator

It is operating in situations such as mud, mold or medical / environment. It may only to defend healthcare staff from germs, by remove at least 95 per cent of small infectious contaminants – unless done properly. This defends against bacteria, not chemicals or vapors.

The 'N' in N95 means that the filter "not resistant to pollution" and 95 means that 95% of the air most penetrating contaminants have been captured by the filter (down to 0.3 microns) through "worst case" testing.

3. P100 gas mask

It protects manual workers from exposure to mercury, asbestos, solvents and other dangerous substances at work. Use in painting/ woodworking; subject them to arsenic; asbestos and solvents.

In comparison, a "P" mask is "oil proof" because this is a kind of overcrowding of a new infection, which is most commonly transmitted by coughing and near communication with men. At least 99,97% of the airborne component is removed by P100 masks, while paper surgical masks do not have nearly the same degree of safety as N95s or N100s due to their loose-fit nature.

4. Full face respirator

Used in painting or situations in which a human needs gas and vapor protection. It covers the skin. It helps in eye defense. It protects gasses and vapors from men. It is most suited for ventilation or vigorous facial hair cases.

5. Self-contained breathing mask

Firefighters use this apparatus. It protects individuals such as firefighters in highly hazardous conditions that need clean air.

Specific recommendations on safekeeping

You will literally breathe in certain diseases. Such are known as diseases in the soil. Airborne disease can transmit if those individuals with illnesses cough, sneeze, or speak, spray nasal and neck secretions into the air. Any viruses or bacteria fly and stay on other humans or objects in the air or on ground.

They take refuge inside of you as you breathe with airborne pathogenic species. This is also possible for you to suck up germs when you touch a surface, and open your own eyes, nose or mouth. These are hard to control because these pathogens fly in the air. Keep thinking on what you should do to safety and understand more about the forms of airborne diseases.

These are hard to control because these pathogens fly in the air. Continue to learn on what you should do to stop yourself from contracting specific kinds of aeronautical diseases.

TYPES OF AIRBORNE DISEASES

1.   THE COMMON COLD

In the United States every year millions of common cold cases occur. Two or three colds a year occur mostly in adults. Children are most likely to have them.

The temperature is the key reason why school and jobs are missing. A lot of viruses will contribute to frost, but it is typically a rhinovirus.

2.   INFLUENZA

Many of them are victims of the flu. It is so quickly infectious that the days you experience the first signs were contagious. In another 5 to 7 days it is infectious. You will extend it to anyone faster than that because you have a compromised immune system for whatever reason.

There are various influenza types, and they change continuously. It makes the production of immunities challenging for the body.

3.   CHICKENPOX

The varicella-zoster virus causes chickenpox. You will disseminate it for a day and two before you get the bluish rash, if you have chickenpox. The illness will grow for up to 21 days following exposure.

Often people just get chickenpox once, and the virus then goes asleep. When the infection is reactivated later in life, the rash is called shingles.

You can get chickenpox from anyone with shingles if you do not have chickenpox.

4.   MUMPS

Mumps is another infectious illness that is very contagious. You should disseminate it before and up to 5 days after symptoms. In the United States, mumps is very widespread, but rates decreased by 99 percent due to vaccination.

70 cases were reported in the United States to the CDC from 1 January to 25 January 2020. Outbreaks are typically found in especially in urban areas.

5.   MEASLES

Measles is a disease that is highly infectious, especially in crowded environments.

The mezzanine virus will continue to work up to 2 hours in the air or on surfaces. Up to 4 days and 4 days before measles rash occurs, you may spread it to others.

Only once do any people having measles.

Measles is the world's leading cause of death for babies, causing 140,000 Trusted Source deaths in 2018. Since 2000 to 2018, the measles vaccine is believed to have stopped around 23 million deaths.

The disease is less prevalent in the USA and occurs more in non-vaccinated individuals. In 2019, 1,282 Authorized Source cases have been registered. Twelve confirmed cases were identified in 2020 by 2 March 2020.

6.   WHOOPING COUGH

This lung disease causes the lung tract to swell which leads to a prolonged cough. It is around 2 weeks after the coughing starts at the point of contagion.

Worldwide, nearly 24.1 million cases of whooping cough are reliable source per year and 160,700 are killed.

There were 15,609 cases reported in the United States in 2018 Reliable Source.

7.   TUBERCULOSIS

Airborne illness is pneumonia, also known as ingestion. This infection is bacterial and does not easily spread. You will typically be in close contact with a person who has it for a long time.

TB may be infected or transferred to others without being sick.

Worldwide, nearly 1.4 billion people have TB. Many are not ill. Some are not ill. Worldwide, nearly 10 million people have TB.

The biggest chance of contracting the disorder is for those with a compromised immune system. Within days of exposure, signs can occur. Some people have to disable for months or years.

Bacteria rapidly increase and invade lungs while the disease becomes involved. This will spread to other tissues, bones or skin through the bloodstream and lymph nodes.

8.   DIPHTHERIA

In the United States, Diphtheria has once been a significant cause of illness and death of babies. Less than five cases have been recorded over the last decade due to universal vaccination.

In 2016, about 7,100 cases were identified diphtheria source worldwide, but may be rarely reported.

The disorder injures and can destroy the liver, kidneys and nerves of the air system.

SYMPTOMS

The following signs are usually caused by respiratory diseases:

- Coughing

- Sneezing

- Runny nose

- Sore throat

- Congestion

- Headache

- Body aches

- Swollen glands

- Loss of appetite

- Fatigue

- Fever

Chickenpox is responsible for an itchy rash which typically begins on your arms, neck, and back before spreading across the rest of your body. In a couple of days, the blisters are fluid-filled. In just a fortnight, the blisters erupted and splashed.

The rash of the measles can take 7 to 18 days after exposure. It usually starts on your face and neck and stretches over a several days. Within a week, it will go ahead.

Significant symptoms of measles include:

- Vomiting
- Dehydration
- Ear infections,
- Severe brain swelling
- Blindness
- Encephalitis

Whooping cough is named for the primary symptom, a prolonged coughing cough, usually accompanied by a heavy air intake.

Symptoms of TB differ according to the organ(s) or the body's processes which may involve secretions or blood coughing.

Diphtheria can induce the neck to swell considerably. It can make breathing and swallowing difficult.

Airborne disease risks are most common for very young people, very old people and those with a compromised immune system.

Anything you do to keep infectious pathogens from spreading?

While airborne infections cannot be totally eliminated, you may do anything to minimize the risk of being sick: avoid direct contact with people who have severe disease symptoms.

- When you are tired, sit put.

- Do not let insecure people touch you in close contact.

- Wear a face mask to avoid transmitting or getting in germs should you choose to be with people.

- When you cough or sneeze, close your mouth. Use your thumb or elbow to reduce the risk for passing germs into your mouth.

- Thoroughly (20 seconds) wash your hands and regularly, particularly after sneezing.

- Stop scratching with unwashed hands your nose or other objects.

Vaccines will reduce the risk of certain airborne diseases. And in the population, vaccines minimize the harm of others.

To cope with all the hazards, the easy and the cheaper way is to wear a face mask and make it. Face mask can easily be made at home.

How to place a face mask and remove it

Usable facial masks can be used once, and then discarded into the garbage. When they are wet, you can always wash and replace masks.

Meet company instructions on mask usage and handling, and protocols for placing on and removing a mask.

PROCEDURE OF REMOVING A FACE MASK

Clean your hands before touching the mask, with soap or water or a hand sanitizer. The mask's front is dirty. Contact the ears / tidies / band only. Follow the following directions for the mask type you use

Ear-looped face mask: hold the ear loops and raise and cover the mask gently.

Ties face mask: First remove the lower arch and then disengage the top arch, then draw the mask away as ties are loosened.

Band face mask: Raise the bottom band over your head and slip the top band over your headfirst.

In the trash dump the mask. Clean your hands with the sanitizer for soap and water or hand.

Chapter 10: Use and Reuse of Medical Masks

Barrier protections such as masks and respirators are seen as the last line of protection against the transmission of bacteria and viruses. Good preventive measures are proven to be effective: vaccination, early warning, isolation and antiviral medicines (as prophylaxis or treatment), and administrative interventions (e.g., banning visitors, informing patients and staff, and confining healthcare workers assigned to an epidemic unit). Key preventive measures, including vaccines and antiviral prophylaxis, may therefore not be available. Public health officials would still need to prescribe respiratory protection in the form of (surgical or procedural) masks, respirators, or both to protect healthcare staff and the public from a virus pandemic, although that may also be problematic if the availability of disposable medical masks although respirators become unsatisfactory. It is allowed that the reuse of masks and respirators intended to be disposable by design changes, cleaning, and decontamination, or other means.

The topic on the use of respiratory protection to manage infectious spread is addressed in this part, explains the problems posed by reuse, examines what is understood about the use of disposable medical masks and respirators in comparable cases, and discusses the implications of reuse of these masks.

Guidance Regarding Use of Surgical Masks

Throughout healthcare settings during times of elevated group activity for respiratory infections, patients with respiratory disease symptoms should be given medical masks as part of a plan for respiratory hygiene. It is recommended that patients wear surgical masks before:

- Symptoms are known not to be triggered by a disease requiring precautions against droplet transmission, or

- A person with symptoms was isolated or put in a room with other patients with the same infection.

It is also advised that medical staff wear masks as part of routine droplet procedures while in close contact with patients with respiratory infection symptoms before or until the patient is found to be non-infectious. Infected adults will transmit the virus until one day before symptoms begin and continue to spread the virus for as long as five days after illness. It is noted that the limited use of masks in non-healthcare settings cannot be adequate for significantly curtailing population transmission. Instead, it advises those with respiratory problems to exercise cough etiquette while they are in another person's presence. The ill people are advised to avoid contact with others and to wear a mask if they cannot.

The Hospital Isolation Precautions Guideline advises that health care staff protect themselves from any airborne illness (airborne transmission) by using a respirator that is at least as safe as a fitted N95 respirator. It is recognized that no controlled trials have tested the efficacy of mask use in preventing virus transmission. Furthermore, personal respiratory protection particulate filter systems capable of filtering at least 95 percent (N95) 0.3 μm particles should be worn at all times while treating patients with suspected or confirmed virus infection.

Guidance on the Reuse of Disposable Equipment and Masks

Most organizations and medical groups advocate the one-time use and recycling of surgical masks and the filtering of face piece respirators, or, at least, that a wearer removes the system when it becomes damp. Medical masks should usually be rotated between applications and whenever damp. It is recommended that surgical masks not be reused during the day or protected by hanging them around the neck or tucking them in a pocket for potential use as the filter part of the mask harbors bacteria gathered from the nasopharyngeal airway, so caution must be taken when removing the mask to prevent contamination of the hands.

Three forms of reuse exist:

a) Among patients with adequate treatment (as with an endoscope),

b) Reuse by the same person with adequate treatment and decontamination (as with contact lenses), and

c) Regular use by the same person over a period of time with or without reprocessing.

The tools or masks are also split into following separate groups:

- Class I apps are for low-risk applications.

- Class II devices are designed for an intermediate level of risk; they require special and general controls.

- Class III products are products at high risk and need pre-market approval.

Masks and respirators are apparatuses in Class II. It is recommended that one patient disposes of medical masks after one use and that healthcare workers donate a new medical mask or respirator any time they come into contact with a new patient. It is also claimed that washing disposable medical masks would degrade their barrier properties, so they will not prevent infection anymore; thus, there is no way to disinfect disposable medical masks.

This must meet the following criteria for a product to be licensed for reuse:

1. The directions shall state the correct micro-biocidal endpoint for the prescribed method of reprocessing.

2. The reprocessing approach must be practical in light of the planned reprocessing location (e.g., hospital versus home use).

3. Instructions for the reprocessing have to be checked.

4. After n number of repeated reprocessing times, the device must still meet the original device's specified performance specifications.

In addition, the design of reusable devices requiring cleaning, disinfection, or sterilization between uses must require the required steps to be adequately performed, and manufacturers must ensure that devices can be effectively reprocessed after repeated use and must create and validate reprocessing procedures.

Manufacturers have claimed that currently manufactured disposable medical masks are made of materials that are likely to deteriorate with normal disinfection levels (e.g., chemicals, heat, and radiation). Since medical masks are intended for disposal, however, it should be remembered that the same user can use a tool again and again until it is damaged, interferes with breathing, or is clearly soiled. Additionally, manufacturers expressed concern that if products built and intended for disposal were recommended for reuse; they would incur increased liability.

It is recommended that healthcare facilities should allow reuse as long as the system is not visibly soiled or damaged (e.g., creased or torn). Reuse will increase the potential for contamination, but this risk must be balanced against the need to provide healthcare workers with maximum respiratory protection. It is also recommended that if disposable N95 respirators are reused for interaction with patients with viruses, healthcare centers will adopt a secure reuse protocol to avoid contamination by touching the outside of the respirator with infectious droplets.

Mask Use Guidelines

The guidelines on the use of masks to allow hospitals and other health centers to stretch resources during this period of high demand. Any of these steps include:

- Remove face masks in public areas for travelers unless they demonstrate signs.

- Extended use of face masks, such as carrying on wearing the same mask when seeing several patients. It is necessary to remember that the mask should be disposed of if it is soiled, dirty, or hard to breathe through. Besides, the wearer cannot reach the mask outside. Wearers can remove the mask only until they are removed from the field of patient care.

- Patients with symptoms use a cloth or other barriers to cover their mouth and nose by using masks.

- Use of masks past the sell-by date of the manufacturer, so long as they are not harmed.

- Cancelation of elective procedures that require face masks.

- Minimal reuse of face masks, where they are removed and placed back on amongst patients seeing. It can be achieved only with masks that are not soiled, broken, or hard to breathe through. In order to prevent contamination, masks should be kept when folded inwards, and tie back masks should not be used for this purpose. Wearers can only remove them until they are removed from the field of patient care.

- Prioritization of the masks for the appropriate activities. This involves required surgeries and procedures when splashes or sprays are likely, for prolonged close contact with potentially infectious patients, or for aerosol-generating procedures if respirators are not available.

Contamination and Reuse of Medical Masks

Respiratory safety schemes, either by the wearer or by the community, will tackle the problem of respiratory pollution. This question is key to concerns about respiratory safety equipment being used again.

Wearer Contamination

In particular, high humidity and temperature within the respirator may lead to microbiological growth in the case of negative-pressure respirators. In general, this problem has been addressed by institutional cleaning and sanitizing policies. Different policies depend on how different people are given respirators or exchanged between users. Respirators should not be reused regularly without washing and should be washed and disinfected until each reassignment when the respirators are used by many individuals.

Filtering face-piece respirators were usually considered disposable due to the inability to clean and disinfect them, although some workplaces allowed the repeated wearing of the same filtering face-piece over a single working day. Additionally, respirators are not deemed "cleanable," although reuse protocols have been introduced during the virus epidemic to resolve shortages. Surgical masks are often considered single-use instruments and are usually discarded following a particular patient treatment or medical procedure mission.

When N95 respirators are reused for patient communication, perform a more reliable reuse procedure to avoid contamination by touching infectious droplets outside the respirator.

a) Consider wearing a loose-fitting cover over your respirator, which does not interfere with fit or seal (e.g., surgical mask, face shield).

b) After entering the patient's room, remove the barrier, and perform hand hygiene. Surgical masks should be discarded; clean and disinfect the face covers.

c) Replace and either hang the respirator in a specified area or put it in a bag. (Consider marking respirators with the username before being used to avoid reuse by another person.)

d) Take caution when putting on the face of a used respirator to ensure a proper fit for respiratory protection and to prevent contact with infectious material that may be present outside the mask.

e) Having removed the respirator on the nose, practice hand hygiene.

f) If using elastomeric (rubber) or powered air-purifying respirators (PAPRs), the reusable components should be washed and disinfected after use, as suggested by the manufacturer. If more than one person uses the half- or full-face-piece elastomeric negative pressure respirators, filters should be swapped between individual users. By using PAPRs, the filters should be removed, following the instructions of the manufacturer. All filters used must be removed in a healthy manner.

g) For certain environments, respiratory safety devices with a filter efficiency of 95 percent or higher may not be available due to supply shortages or other factors.

h) In this case, it should wear a surgical (procedural) mask. Surgical masks can provide barrier protection against large droplets, which are considered the primary route of transmission of viruses. Nevertheless, surgical masks cannot adequately protect against airborne particles or aerosols, largely because they require leakage across the mask and cannot be checked to match. The mask can withstand penetration of the fluid and fit securely around the mouth and nose when applied correctly to the face.

i) In all encounters with suspect patients or items that may be infected with the virus, including handwashing with soap and water, hand hygiene is urged; if hands are not clearly soiled, hand rubbing based on alcohol can be used as an alternative to hand washing.

Environmental Contamination

Exposure to airborne pollutants can also contribute to contamination of the respirator or medical mask's surface as well as to filter material contamination. Environmental contamination can result from the deposition of toxic (chemical or biological) substances on the respirator body or surgical mask. It can, for example, happen in an industrial setting when the respirator is worn in a dusty atmosphere. In a medical environment, an example of infection is the distribution of infectious particles around an infected patient who is coughing or sneezing. This form of infection is of particular concern because the material or species may reach the body after handling (e.g., through skin absorption, ingestion, or interaction with mucous membranes).

In fact, the filter pollution applies to the accumulation of species on filters (in the case of exposures to aerosols). Laboratory loading studies of inert bacterial particles have shown that although filters catch particles in the media, they retain particles with considerable attractive force and are very difficult to extract, particularly when the filter is exposed to large airbursts similar to coughs and sneezes or when dropped onto a hard surface. As a consequence, the filter material does not pose a threat during the use of respirators and medical masks.

Nevertheless, it is likely that heavily loaded filters can release particles during handling since weaker attractive forces can retain the particles. The details on the medical masks are much less definitive. In the event of an outbreak, fit can have a great effect on effectiveness, and usage procedures, including place of use, are likely to also be significant factors.

The disposable medical masks and respirators have not been built for reuse, and there is almost universal consensus that reuse should be avoided, even by a single person, except in the most severe and desperate circumstances.

Enjoying this book?

Please leave a review because we would love to hear your feedback, opinions and advice to create better products and services for you! Thank you for your support. You are greatly appreciated!"

Chapter 11: For Emergency, What We Should Do?

Using Clothes (Scarf, Bandana, etc.)

This method is meant for single wear only. After one use, you should take the clothes off carefully and wash them with a disinfecting agent, then either wash your hands with soap or sanitize your hands.

Protection level: up to 20%

Where to use home, empty street

Wearing time: up to 1-2 hours

If you need to go out but you have no suitable mask with you — use wearable items, like a scarf or bandana.

Paper Towels

Attention! This mask is meant for single use only. After one use, you need to take it off carefully and throw away, then either wash your hands with soap or sanitize your hands.

Protection level: up to 20%

Where to use home, empty street

Wearing time: up to 5-30 minutes (the mask can quickly become wet, which dramatically decreases its ability to protect you)

Three-layer masks and four-layer masks of towels are the most efficient.

Materials:

- Paper towels or napkins
- 2 rubber bands

- Stapler

STEP 1. Tear a paper hand towel off a roll and fold it like an accordion.

STEP 2. Fold the paper in a single strip and place the rubber bands onto its ends.

STEP 3. Fold the paper end to cover the rubber band and secure it with a stapler on both sides.

The mask is ready! Now, all you need to do is to smooth out its middle part and put it on your face, covering all airways.

You can do the same by replacing paper towels with a piece of cloth; see the example below.

Face Tissue

This method is meant for single wear only. After one use, you should take the mask off carefully and wash it with a disinfecting agent, then either wash your hands with soap or sanitize your hands.

Protection level: up to 20%

Where to use home, empty street

Wearing time: up to 1-2 hours

Materials:

- Bandana (or square cotton cloth approximately 20" x 20")

- Rubber bands (or hair ties)

- Scissors (if you cut your clothing)

Quick Cut T-Shirt Face Covering

This method is meant for single wear only. After one use, you should take the mask off carefully and wash it with a disinfecting agent, then either wash your hands with soap or sanitize your hands.

Protection level: up to 20%

Where to use home, empty street

Wearing time: up to 1-2 hours

Materials:

- T-shirt (or any other suitable clothing)
- Scissors

Gauze masks

Gauze masks offer the simplest form of protection. They are often used for medical purposes in the absence of direct contact with patients. It protects against strong smells and copes rather well with a low concentration of caustic substances.

This type of mask is rarely used nowadays, as this method is believed to be outdated. However, properly disinfected gauze can withstand repeated use, and it is easy to treat it with radio and quartz sterilizers, boiling water and simple disinfecting solutions.

Reusable Gauze Masks for Kids and Adults

The fact that this mask is reusable does not mean that it can be used all day long. It is meant to be worn for 2-3 hours. After being used, the item should be washed with soap, treated with antiseptic, dried, and then ironed.

Protection level: up to 40%

Where to use home, street, shop

Wearing time: up to 2 hours

You need a sewing kit to create this mask.

Materials:

- Medical gauze
- Template
- Needle with thread
- Scissors
- Tape measure

Detailed Description of a 6-8-Layer Mask for Kids:

Such protective means can be made not only for children but for adults as well, considering individual sizes.

STEP 1: If you want to protect your child, we recommended sewing a mask to particular sizes. You will need two parameters — length and width. You should measure the length with a tape measure. First place it at on ear. Then, lay it across the nose to the second ear.

STEP 2: To measure the width, place the tape to the middle of the nose. Lay it downward across the nose and mouth to the middle of the chin.

Step 3: Write down the sizes, add 1 to 1.5 inches for allowances and cut the template out of paper. Make 3-4 layers of gauze. Attach the template and cut out a rectangle. You will need 2 such rectangles.

Step 4: Fold the gauze edges from every side and iron them. The rectangles should fit the face size.

Step 5: You will need straps to fix the mask on the face. You can make them using common underwear or anything else with an elastic band. To determine the length of the strap, you should try them on and add 0.5 inches to the resulting size. Straps for a kids' mask should be about 5-6 inches long.

Step 6: Sew the rubber band ends to the corners of one of the gauze blanks. You should do this on both sides.

Step 7: Then cover the blank with elastic bands with the other half (second rectangle blank) and sew along all the sides. Using a sewing machine can help speed up the process.

Usually, 6-8 layers of gauze are enough to protect from infections if the material density fits with the standard. The optimal density of medical gauze should be 36 g/square meter. It can be lower, but by no more than 5%. You can easily check it using scales. If the density is less, you should make a more layered mask (10-20).

Be aware that if the mask is too tight, it can shut off the airways. This is highly dangerous for children and elderly people, as it can result in loss of consciousness. Therefore, you should look for a middle-ground between protection and enabling an ability to breathe freely.

Disposable Cotton Wool and Gauze Mask (No-Sew Method)

After one use, you need to take it off carefully and throw away, then either wash your hands with soap or sanitize your hands.

Protection level: up to 60%

Where to use home, street, shop

Wearing time: up to 4 hours

Instructions:

STEP 1. If the material is loose, make 2 layers.

STEP 2. Flatten the cotton wool and spread it to the middle of the gauze.

STEP 3. Close the cotton wool by rolling it into the gauze up and down.

STEP 4. Cut on either side of the gauze with scissors.

STEP 5. The mask should cover your nose and mouth and reach cheeks up to the ears.

Such a mask is disposable, but it has an advantage. Whereas pharmacy masks must be changed every 2 hours, this gauze-cotton mask can be worn for 3-4 hours.

Disposable Cotton Wool and Gauze Mask (Sew Method)

Protection level: up to 60%

Where to use home, street, shop

Wearing time: up to 4 hours

Attention! This mask is meant for single wear only. After one use, you need to take it off carefully and throw it away, then wash your hands with soap or sanitize your hands.

Materials:

- Sterile gauze, 5,5" wide

- Roll of sterile cotton wool

- White thread

- Common needle for hand sewing

- Scissors

How to do:

STEP 1. Measure out a 24"-long gauze piece and cut it off. It does not make sense to cut off less. (The picture shows measurement in centimeters.)

STEP 2. Fold this bandage piece in half, 4 times, and cut into 2 parts in the middle. These will make up the straps.

STEP 3. Now let us take the cotton wool. Measure out a 5.5"-long cotton wool piece. (The picture shows measurement in centimeters.) We recommend taking a cotton wool roll, which is easy to unroll.

STEP 4. Unfold the gauze and spread the cotton wool over it, leaving a little space from the edge. Those pieces of gauze that we cut off at the very beginning will make up the straps. First, we place one at the first edge. Fold the gauze edge and smooth it with your hand.

STEP 5. Now do the same at the other side with the second gauze piece, which will make up the second strap as well.

STEP 6. Wrap the whole construction with a gauze. You should do this 4 times to get 2 layers on the top and 2 layers on the bottom.

STEP 7. Cut off the excess gauze. Now, let us get down to sewing our mask, so that it does not fall apart.

After sewing the gauze edges, you should iron it on both sides. Only after this step will the mask be ready to use. The result? A homemade, reliable and simple mask that will protect you from coronavirus.

Such a mask is positioned as disposable, but it has an advantage: whereas pharmacy masks need to be changed every 2 hours, this gauze-cotton mask can be worn for 3-4 hours.

Chapter 12: Top 5 DIY Alternative Face Masks

As a last resort, you can turn to alternative solutions that, while not being nearly as effective as those presented in the previous parts, give you some degree of protection against microbes. Keep in mind some masks aren't recommended to use regularly, but only in case of emergencies, and when you're visiting locations that are lower risk and don't include being near other people. For example, this includes leaving the home briefly to walk your pet, empty the trash, or take a short ride to bring essentials over to someone who is in isolation. In this case, if you won't be in close contact with other individuals, and you don't have better solutions, these creative alternatives will be better than not having protection at all.

An Improvised Cloth Mask

If you must improvise a cloth face mask, any larger piece of cotton will do. Items like T-shirt, small, thin dishcloths or towels, when layered and tied around your face, can be a considerable means of protection. Simply grab your large piece of cloth and fold it over as many times as possible to retain the size needed for tying around your head into a rectangular shape. Tuck the middle of the folded piece, place it over your mouth and nose, and tie the corners at the back of your head, below the ears. Tie snugly, but not tight. Repeat the process with the remaining top corners of the folded piece, again making sure that you're tying it snug but not tightly. If your piece is large enough, you'll probably be left with some extra fabric on the sides of your face, under your chin, and over your nose. Tuck these ends in to seal the gaps, but without further constricting your nose and mouth. Tuck and adjust until you feel like you're breathing only through the fabric, without air coming in from the sides of the mask. The effectiveness of this mask increases with the number of layers, so make sure to apply the maximum number of layers that still allow you to breathe properly.

Plastic Sheeting Shield Mask

The use of plastic on your face, and particularly improvising a shield, is questionable without any doubt. However, if you're in a high-risk situation and your contact with the possible infection will last only briefly, this is an acceptable alternative in case you don't have an original, quality face shield. For this mask alternative, you will need a piece of plastic sheeting in 12-inch length. You will also need some foam tape or weather stripping, or electrical tape that's around ½-inch or ¾-inch wide. You will also need a pair of flat shoelaces, a stapler, and a hole punch.

First, cut the sheeting into a piece that's 12 inches long and 8 ½ inches wide. Cut 12 inches of either weather stripping or foam tape and apply it to the upper edge of the plastic. Apply pieces of electrical tape on the sides of the plastic sheet, folding over the edges to dull the edges of the sheet. Use either a stapler or the punch to pierce holes in the top corners of the shield, where you apply the foam tape, and pull one shoelace on each side, leaving enough length for tying on the back of your head. Staple the shoelaces to keep them in place. Before putting on your plastic face shield, carefully disinfect both inside and outside while wearing gloves. Make sure that your shield is fully dry before putting it on.

Snorkeling Goggles

Got spare snorkeling goggles from your last vacation? They can help in protecting against catching other people's droplets. Snorkeling goggles and masks have also been used as an alternative and the last resort in the line of the fight against contagious diseases. If you're compelled to leave your home and visit a potentially crowded area, and you don't have a reliable mask by your side, snorkeling goggles and mask can be an effective alternative.

Scuba Face Masks

Scuba face masks are often referred to as a last resort in protection against catching contagious droplets. While they might be effective in disallowing droplets to fall onto your nose and mouth, they are still constricting in terms of breathing, and may not be suitable for those with chronic respiratory problems. If you must, you can wear a scuba face mask on your way out, but only briefly and with proper sanitation. While wearing gloves, sanitize the mask both inside and out and wait for it to dry completely. Before putting the mask on, wash both your hands and your face.

Wet Wipe Mask

Last in the line of alternatives to improvise a face mask when you don't have any better solutions is to use a wet wipe. Antibacterial wet wipes (supposedly) kill off germs before they can reach your respiratory tract. These claims have been debunked by scientific researchers, but the notion that any protection is better than no protection at all prevailed when including this idea into the book.

How to make a wet wipe face mask? If you must do this, we recommend choosing an antibacterial wipe, because these contain disinfectants. Preferably, the wipes should be of the highest quality and large enough to cover your face without stretching. Use your fingers or sharp tools to pierce larger holes near the sides of the wet wipe, making sure that the location of the holes allows snug-but-not-tight placing. When you've pierced the holes in the wet wipe, simply apply your makeshift mask by putting it over your face, grabbing the edge of the sides to widen the holes to go over your ears, and attaching the edges at the back of your ears.

With the notion that this design is as ineffective as DIYs can get, we recommend using only for low-risk outside errands, or as an extra layer of protection underneath your other DIY solutions, like when you're improvising a face mask with cotton pieces of fabric.

Chapter 13: Homemade Face Shield and Improvised Gas Mask

Face masks are recommended for curbing the spread of the virus because they help to cover the nose and mouth so that droplets will not escape and infect others. But, face shields are even better than the masks because they provide overall protection for the face, not only the nose and mouth. The face shields are also durable and last longer.

Also, unlike surgical masks that are usually reusable, face shields are reusable because they can be cleaned after use. When you face masks of any type, there is a high probability that you will touch your face, thereby get infected, but with the face shield, your face is completely isolated, and you can't feel it. The face shield is more natural to communicate since the mouth is not covered but protected, and you can breathe easily. Face shields are very comfortable.

Homemade Face Shield

Materials

•1 long transparent flat plastic folder

•1 small face towel or cotton fabric

•1 elastic tie or string

•Scissors

•Pen

•Ruler

•Puncher

•Any circular object like tape, cup.

•Glue

•Decorative tape

•Cardboard

Direction

•Cut the cardboard and glue it to the top of the flat plastic transparent folder.

•Place the transparent plastic on a flat surface

•Pick the circular object and place it on the bottom edge of the transparent flat plastic.

•Use a scissor to cut out the edges of the plastic to give it a curved edge.

•Pick the puncher, use it to punch holes on the sides of the top of the glued cardboard.

•Place the face towel on the cardboard edge to fit the length.

•Fold the sheet four times from the top, and cut away the remaining part.

•Unfold the towel and put glue at the middle, and fold together again.

• Put some glue on the cardboard and place the glued towel against it to hold it in place.

•Put your decorative tape over the edges of the plastic. Use the scissor to make incisions on the rugged edges to smoothen it over. Put the decorative tape over the cardboard too.

•Take the strings and insert them in the holes on the cardboard. Tie the ends to a knot.

• The plastic should be curved now and ready to wear.

The gas mask is not a medical mask, but it is effective against viruses and organisms that reside in the air. It is also useful when someone you are trapped in an unclean, corrupt, and polluted environment. The gas mask is effective against the Virus because of recent reports that the Virus can also be spread through farts. If an infected individual fart, another person that inhales the fart is at risk of getting infected. This is because the Virus also resides in digestive tracts and is still alive on excretes. Furthermore, the gas mask covers the entire face, not only the nose and mouth.

Getting a gas mask usually costs hundreds of dollars; in this DIY method, we'll be making a gas with regular home materials that you can get even without going out. Making this gas mask is tricky because all its parts must be correctly fixed together, or you stand a risk of inhaling lousy air.

Materials

For one person

•2-liter soda bottle or any bottle

•1 Dust mask

•Knife

Direction

•Get the 2-liter bottle, trim, and cut with a knife through the seam you find under the bottle. Cut off the bottom completely.

• Remove the label from the plastic. Use the knife to cut a U-shape around the area where the remaining label is.

• Make a 2-inches cut in a U-shape above the cap of the bottle.

•Cut the width of the U-shape to fit perfectly on your face. Don't make it too big to avoid gas or droplets getting into it.

•Pick your dusk mask, remove the bands from it, and set aside.

•Pick the cut bottle, stuff the dust mask into it. Tilt the mask a bit down towards the bottle cap to create a small chamber between the mask and the cap.

• Get the duct tape, use it to hold down and secure the mask firmly to the bottle. Ensure that you have a solid seal around the mask—no gaps to avoid bad air sneaking in.

•After cutting and making the shape on the bottle, you'll have jagged edges. To close off these edges, use the duct tape to surround the edges to make it more comfortable. When you put duct tape on the edges, it allows the bottle to fit well, and you get a better seal around the face.

• On the edges of the bottle, cut some slits into it. Insert the mask bands into it. Make one slit on each side of the bottle near the top. Measure four inches below the first slits, make another slit again.

• Insert the bands through the slit and thread. Thread from the inside of the bottle and thread out. Make an overhand knot of the band outside and tie off.

• Cover the slits and bands with duct tapes to prevent air from gaining entry through there. This will also serve as added security for the bands.

• Use the knife to punch holes or make a small square shape in the bottle to allow adequate air intake.

• Place and fit on your face. Make adjustments where necessary, and that's all!

How to wear and remove a disposable respirator

Due to the sensitivity of Virus, it is important to educate you on how to wear different types of face masks.

You must be wearing the masks correctly.

The following are the simple steps involved with wearing and removing the disposable respirator mask.

First, let me mention that if you have used a respirator before and it fits perfectly, it is good to get that same model, size, and make.

Also, before you put the respirator on your face, it is vital to inspect it for any damages. If you notice any damage to it, DO NOT USE IT.

For proper placement of the mask, remove any impediments like facial hair, jewelry, glasses, etc.

To put on the respirator,

• Position the respirator properly in your hand with the nose piece resting on your fingertips.

• Cup the respirator, allowing the headbands to hang below your hand and hold it under your chin with the nosepiece up.

• The top strap goes over the top back of your head while the bottom strap goes around the neck and below the ears.

• If there is a metal nose clip on the respirator, place your fingertips from both hands on it and slide down to mold the metal clip around the nose.

To check if the seal of the respirator is working properly

• Cover the respirator and take a quick breath in to check the seal is tightly placed on the face.

• Place both hands on the respirator entirely and breathe out. If you feel air leakage on your hands, that means there is no proper seal on the respirator.

• If the air leakage is around the nose, re-adjust the nosepiece. If the leakage is from the edge of the mask, re-adjust the straps along the sides of the head until it is properly sealed.

•If, after readjustments, you still feel leakages and cannot achieve a proper seal, try on a different mask size or model.

To remove the respirator from your face.

•DO NOT TOUCH the respirator at the front as it may be contaminated.

•Remove the respirator by pulling the bottom strap over the back of the head. Then, pull the top strap. Do these without touching the respirator.

•Discard the respirator and wash your hands.

Conclusion

Think about all the things you have touched today: papers, raw food, objects, money, animals etc. Whatever it is, you have surely come into contact with germs and your hands, especially around your nails, are one of your favorite places to stay. Washing your hands frequently and correctly can eliminate them. Furthermore, if you neglect the hygiene of your hands, especially when you are sick, you will spread germs in your path, and they will stay on other people or on surfaces that others will then touch. In fact, this is one of the main ways of spreading the cold or the flu, for example. So there is no doubt that hand washing is the first line of defense against germs

The skin is not only our natural envelope; it also acts as a barrier that prevents the passage of germs to our body. These are just some tips that you can follow to take care of it: protect it from the sun, avoid continual rubbing of the skin with clothing and footwear to avoid chafing and infections and make sure that it is always dry, because with moisture the skin is macerated and loses its barrier capacity against infections. After showering, carefully dry your entire body. A tip: if you can dry clothes in the sun, this will eliminate many microbe

As you can see, making your own face masks is a great idea especially in times of turmoil. We hope that this guide has been useful in getting you the information you need to make your own masks. After all, the health and wellbeing of you and your loved ones are at stake here. So, there is no need to take any chances when you can have everything covered and firmly in control.

Thank you very much for taking the time to read this guide on how to make your own homemade medical face masks. In times of crisis, it is always good to know that you are ready in case anything should happen. That is why making your own masks can give you the peace of mind in knowing that you will not have to panic when there are shortages of medical supplies.

In addition, making your own masks ensures that you are using quality materials that you know will help protect your family. While a homemade mask is not as effective as a professional-grade respirator, the fact of the matter is you have the protection that can keep you safe during a crisis. Plus, having your own masks can help you stay protected even when you may have professional-grade masks on hand.

Please take the time to network this information to everyone you think would benefit from it. They will surely find it useful to know how to make their own medical face masks. The more people able to do make their own masks, the better protected our communities will be. So, please tell them about this book. If possible, help others make their own masks. That way, you can also become a teacher in your neighborhood and in your community.

So, thanks again for taking the time to read this book. We hope it has been as useful and informative as we hope it has been. This information has worked for countless families. It will hopefully work for yours, too.

Finally, if you found this book useful in any way, a review on Amazon is always appreciated!

Diy Homemade Hand Sanitizer:

A Complete Step By Step Guide To Fight Germ And Bacteria With Alcohol-Based And Natural Recipes. Learn How To Make Your Own Hand Sanitizer And Home Disinfectant

Gabriel Blakely

Introduction

As the old cliché goes, cleanliness is next to godliness. You might have already encountered this old adage numerous times in your life. You might have even used it yourself. But have you ever really taken the time to just sit down and think about what that means? When you see this saying at first glance, you might be taken aback by its hyperbole. What do they mean when they say that being clean is practically also being godlike? Does making sure that the floors of your bedroom are free of dust mean that you are inching closer to becoming godly?

When you think of a godly entity, you think of something that is invulnerable, invincible, impregnable, indestructible, and all of the other descriptors of that nature. You think of something or someone that would never be brought down by illnesses, disease, and physical ailments. On that note, the old adage starts to make sense now. One of the best ways to make sure that you are not subjecting yourself to harmful germs, bacteria, and viruses is making efforts to stay clean and sanitized. The more exposed you are to these harmful germs and viruses, the more susceptible you will be to becoming ill and weak.

You owe it to yourself to always try to stay healthy and fit. That is the only way that you would ever be able to get everything out of your life that you want. With that, it should be in your best interests that you put forth efforts to always stay clean and sanitary. Not too many people realize that the proper scrubbing of your hands is one of the most effective methods of keeping yourself clean. By simply rubbing your hands with a proper cleaning solution, you will be able to protect yourself from all sorts of germs and viruses. Not only that but keeping yourself clean and free from viruses will mean that those who are around you a lot of the time will be safe as well. On the base level, you want to make sure that any germs or viruses do not compromise your system. But on top of that, you do not want to serve as a carrier for these potentially dangerous viruses for the people you love as well.

To be quite blunt about it, nothing is going to beat the effectiveness of washing your hands with soap. This is why doctors and surgeons always "scrub in" prior to performing any medical procedures. This is the only way that they can make sure that they are sanitized. They need to go through such sanitary measures to protect their patients from any viral or bacterial contaminations. So, if you are really looking to keep yourself clean and sanitary, wash your hands properly and regularly. It is not just a matter of merely getting your hands wet and putting some soap on them. You need to really be thorough in making sure that the cleansing soap gets to every part of your hand's surface area.

However, the problem is that soap and water are not always going to be accessible to everyone. Think about when you are on your morning commute to work. You might take a bus or a train during your journey. Along the way, you are forced to touch so many objects that other people have been touching as well. Door handles. Ticket vending machines. When you get to your office building, you might have to take the elevator up to your floor or you see a workmate along the way. You shake hands. You touch the elevator buttons. All of these micro-interactions that your hand has with everyday objects exposes you to a variety of different germs and bacteria. And it is not like you get an opportunity to wash your hands within that span, right? This is exactly the kind of situation in which a cleaning solution such as rubbing alcohol, or a hand sanitizer would come in handy.

Out of any other body part, your hands are the most susceptible when it comes to the picking up or gathering of different germs or bacteria. This is because the hand is one of the most mechanically functional parts of the human body. You use it for all sorts of purposes in many different scenarios. You use your hands to pick up cell phones, greet other people, and open doors. You also use your hands to scratch your face, to eat your food, or to blow your nose. When you put your hands very close to your nose or mouth like this, you are enabling the quicker transfer of germs and bacteria from the outside world into your system. These germs can potentially overwhelm your body to the point that your immune system becomes compromised and your organs fail to function properly.

The fact of the matter is that your hands need to be protected all the time. And while handwashing is the best method for achieving that, it is not just always going to be possible all throughout the day. You need a more convenient and effective way to still keep your hands clean even when you are on the go. This is why hand sanitizers make for really great everyday essentials that you should have with you at all times. However, getting access to a hand sanitizer or a rubbing alcohol that suits your personal needs is not always going to be easy.

As you may well be aware, in times of major public health crises, items such as rubbing alcohols and hand sanitizers become such precious commodities. As a result, the demand might even start eclipsing the supply. In those cases, you become reliant on the capacity of these manufacturers to increase their production rates so that you get better chances of getting your own disinfectants and sanitary solutions.

But that has not the only problem that people generally have with sanitizing gels and rubbing alcohols that are commercially made. Sometimes, there are people who just do not develop certain affinities toward commercially made hand sanitizers. Some of them say that certain hand sanitizers are too drying and bad for their skin. Others might complain of the overwhelming fragrances that are being emitted by certain brands and products. Also, unbeknownst to a lot of people, there are some sanitizers, air fresheners, and cleaners that may contain certain harmful chemicals as well. The best way to free yourself from these issues would be to directly oversee the manufacturing process of these cleaners and disinfectants yourself.

The biggest problem here is that people think they have to live with their frustrations and be content with the situation. However, that does not necessarily have to be the case. You do not have to be overly reliant on whatever the market can provide you. Sometimes, the best alcohol solution is the one that you come up with on your own. And you should not be intimidated by the process that is involved in making your own hand sanitizer or rubbing alcohol. It really is not all that complicated of a process. In fact, if you have any experience in the kitchen with cooking or at the bar with drinks, it is much like that. It is merely a matter of following certain recipes and making sure that all conditions are satisfied.

This is exactly what this book will help you do. It is okay if you have developed a certain reliance on commercialism for your every needs and utilities. That has just the way that the world is currently laid out. Everything is designed for it to be as convenient and as easy as possible for you. However, there is still definite value in having the knowledge and tools necessary to make things on your own. This book is loaded with all sorts of recipes for cleaning alcohol and hand sanitizers to suit your every need. Some of these recipes will be a lot easier to make, and some will have ingredients that are more difficult to obtain or source. Whatever the case, each recipe is going to have its own defining characteristic, and you are free to use any of them.

Chapter 1: List of Alcohols with Disinfectant Properties

CDC advises that you use alcohol of at least 60 percent in making your hand sanitizer and a minimum of 70 percent alcohol content when making your disinfectant sprays and wipes. Here are alcohols that meet this guideline. 70%+ ethanol products: minimum of 140 proof and above drinkable grain alcohols like:

- Spiritus vodka – 192 proof, 96 percent alcohol

- Golden grain – 190 proof, 95 percent alcohol

- Ever clear – 190 proof, 92.4 percent ethanol
2. 70%+ rubbing alcohol, also called isopropyl alcohol:

- 99% rubbing alcohol

- 91% rubbing alcohol

- 70% rubbing alcohol

Essential Oils with Disinfecting Properties

Here are essential oils that are antiviral, antibacterial, antiseptic, antifungal, antimicrobial, and deodorizing. You can use any of these essential oils in making your disinfectant spray, wipes and hand sanitizer:

- Rosemary
- Lavender
- Orange
- Thyme
- Tea tree
- Geranium
- Clove
- Lemon
- Eucalyptus
- Cinnamon
- Chamomile
- Thieves blend
- Basil oil

Essential Oil	Properties
Geranium	Antiviral, antifungal, antibacterial, and antiseptic
Rosemary	antifungal, antibacterial, antiseptic, and antimicrobial
Peppermint	Antiviral, antifungal, antibacterial, antiseptic, and antimicrobial
Lavender essential oil	Antiviral, antifungal, antibacterial, antiseptic, and antimicrobial
Tea tree essential oil	Antiviral, antifungal, antibacterial, antiseptic, and antimicrobial
Orange	Antiviral, antifungal, and antiseptic
Lemon	Antiviral, antifungal, antiseptic, and antimicrobial
Eucalyptus	Antiviral, antifungal, antibacterial, antiseptic, and antimicrobial
Clove	Antiviral, antifungal, antibacterial, and antiseptic

Cinnamon	Antiviral, antifungal, antibacterial, antiseptic, and antimicrobial
Thyme	Antiviral, antibacterial, and antiseptic

Let us now look at the different ways to make your own disinfectants and hand sanitizer:

Homemade Antibacterial Wipes Recipes

Tools Needed

1. Glass bowl
2. Measuring cup

Glass spray bottle

You can use this wipe to clean and disinfectant the following:

- Toddler's hands and face after eating
- Fridge
- Stovetop
- Floor spills
- Dusting
- Light switches
- Benchtops
- Clean taps
- Sink
- Skirting boards
- Microwave
- Taps
- Wall
- And lots more

Here are the different parts of your home you can use these disinfectant wipes on:

Around Your Home

- Doorknobs
- Thermometers
- Phones
- Light switches
- Computer mouse
- Remote controls

Bathroom

- Countertop
- Toilet

- Doorknobs
- Faucets
- Light switches

Kitchen

- Oven handle and knobs
- Countertop
- Refrigerator handles
- Trashcan
- Light switches
- Faucet
- Cabinet pulls

Outside My Home

- Restaurant table
- Shopping cart
- Gearshift and steering wheel in your car

Tips for Choosing Wipe Container

1. You need a container that can hold at least thirty to forty paper towels and the disinfectant solution.

2. Whatever container you choose should be able to accommodate the essential oils. Note that essential oils can damage some plastic containers. So, it is advisable to go for stainless steel, glass, and a few plastics that are compatible with essential oils.

3. Your container also needs to have an airtight lid to stop the wipes from drying off.

Here are some containers that you can use to store your homemade wipes:

- Glass mason jars
- An old wipes container

- Clean plastic food containers

- Cereal storage containers

- A gallon-sized or quart jar with plastic lid

Tips for Choosing Material for Your Wipes

You can make use of paper towels like the single-ply ones sold in the dollar stores. You can also use square cuts from lint-free towels or old white t-shirts that you can always wash and re-use.

Let us now look at all the various wipe recipes.

All-Purpose Cleaning Disinfectant Wipes

Total Time: 3 min

Ingredients

- Warm water – 2 cups
- Liquid soap – 1 tablespoon
- 70%+ rubbing alcohol – 1 cup
- Lemon essential oil – 10 drops
- Paper towel – 1

Instructions

1. Add all the liquid in a bowl. Mix together.

2. Place one roll of paper towel in a large rectangular container or an old wipe container.

3. Pour the liquid over the paper towels.

4. Cover with the lid and shake until the towels are well saturated.

5. Pull out the cardboard tube from the paper towels.

6. Use the wipes when needed

Reusable Antibacterial Wipes

Total Time: 3 min

Ingredients

- Rubbing alcohol – 1 cup
- Water – 1 cup
- Lavender oil – 12 drops
- Peppermint oil (or your preferred oil) – 5 drops
- Microfiber cloths
- Detergent – 2 teaspoons
- Large airtight container

Instructions

1. Cut the towels into square sizes and add them into a large container or an old wipes container.

2. Mix all the remaining ingredients in a bowl

3. Pour the mixture over the cloth.

4. Seal the container.

5. Shake the container to get the cloth wet with the mixture.

6. Use when needed, wash once used/ dirty.

DIY Homemade Clorox Wipes

Total Time: 3 min

Ingredients

- Water – ½ cup
- 99% rubbing alcohol or 95% ethanol – ½ cup
- Hydrogen peroxide – 2 tablespoons
- Paper towels – ½ roll
- Basil essential oil – 15 drops
- Lemon essential oil – 10 drops
- Tea tree essential oil – 20 drops

Instructions

1. Cut one paper towel roll into two equal sizes.

2. Take one half of the paper towel and place it in a large container.

3. Mix all the remaining ingredients into a bowl.

4. Pour the mixture over the cloth.

5. Seal the container.

6. Shake the container to get the cloth wet with the mixture.

7. Now pull out the cardboard insert.

8. Use a Pin to drill a hole on the container lid so that you can easily pull out the center paper towel.

9. Use when needed.

Disinfectant Lysol Wipes for Hard Surfaces

Total Time: 3 min

Ingredients

- Washcloths – 10
- Dawn dishwashing soap – 3 teaspoons
- 70%+ rubbing alcohol – 2 cups
- Basil essential oil – 10 drops

Instructions

1. Cut the washcloths into square sizes or in halves.

2. Add the washcloths to your container or jar

3. Mix all the remaining ingredients in a bowl.

4. Pour the liquid mixture over the washcloths.

5. Cover with a lid and shake vigorously.

6. Use as needed. Wash in the laundry when dirty.

Homemade Disinfecting Wipes

Total Time: 3 min

Ingredients

- 70%+ rubbing alcohol – 3 cups
- 3% Hydrogen peroxide – ¾ teaspoon
- Tea tree essential oil – 20 drops
- Clove essential oil – 15 drops
- Cinnamon bark essential oil – 10 drops
- Rosemary essential oil – 5 drops
- Eucalyptus essential oil - 5 drops
- Paper towels or washcloths

Instructions

1. Add the alcohol, hydrogen peroxide, and the oils into a cup or bowl. Mix together.

2. Pour two cups of the mixture into your wipe container.

3. Get your paper towels, disposable guest towels, or even an old white cloth. If using a piece of fabric, cut into square sizes. Then fold each of the towels or cloth in half. Arrange the towels or cloth on top of each other.

4. Fold the stacked wipes in two then place them into the container.

5. Cover the container and shake it well to get the towels well soaked in the liquid.

6. Pour the remaining liquid over the wipes. Shake again.

7. Then set aside to use when needed. Wash the cloth wipes in the laundry when used.

6. Homemade Lysol Wipes

Total Time: 3 min

Ingredients

- 70%+ rubbing alcohol – ¼ cup
- Water – 1 cup
- Dawn dish soap – 1 teaspoon
- Ammonia – 2 tablespoons
- Washcloths – 24

Instructions

1. Cut the washcloths into square sizes and add them to a large jar or container.

2. Mix the remaining ingredients in a bowl.

3. Then pour the liquid over the content of the wipe container.

4. Cover with a lid and shake vigorously

5. Use as needed. Wash in the laundry when dirty.

Homemade Bathroom and Kitchen Cleaning Wipes

Total Time: 3 min

Ingredients

- Distilled water – ¾ cup
- White vinegar – ¼ cup
- Liquid castile soap – ½ teaspoon (unscented)
- Thyme oil – 10 drops
- Tea tree essential oil – 10 drops
- Sweet orange – 10 drops
- Paper towels – 30

Instructions

1. You can also use paper napkins, disposable guest towels, or old clean cloth to replace the paper towels. If using fabric, cut into square sizes.

2. Mix all the liquid ingredients in a glass container.

3. Shake gently to mix your ingredients.

4. Roll up the towels then place them in your glass jar.

5. Cover the jar and shake gently to get the wipes well saturated.

6. Use for all your cleaning needs.

Simple Homemade Hand Wipes

Total Time: 3 min

Ingredients

- Dish soap - 1 tablespoon
- Warm water - 2 cups
- 70%+ rubbing alcohol - 1 cup
- Half a roll of paper towels
- Tupperware container

Instructions

1. Mix all the liquid ingredients in a glass bowl.

2. Place the paper towels in your Tupperware container, then pour the liquid mixture over the paper towels

3. Shake the bottle well to get the towels wet with the liquid.

4. You may replace the paper towels with your washcloth or old fabric. Wash thoroughly after each use.

Natural Lysol Disinfectant Wipes

Total Time: 3 min

Ingredients

- White Distilled Vinegar - 1 Cup
- Small washcloths or Pre-Cut Cloth - 20 Pieces
- Filtered Water - 1 Cup
- Tea Tree Essential Oil - 8 Drops
- Bergamot Essential Oil - 4 Drops
- Lemon Essential Oil - 15 Drops

Instructions

1. Add all the liquid ingredients in a glass mason jar.

2. Cover and shake to mix the ingredients.

3. Soak the cloths in the liquid. Shake the jar until the wipes are well saturated.

4. Store and use when needed.

5. Wash the wipes when used or dirty.

How to Use

1. Whenever you need to use the disinfectant wipe, simply pull out one cloth, squeeze out the excess liquid, then use the wipes on your porcelain, linoleum, glass, tile or stain less steel surface.

2. Wash used wipes in the laundry.

Homemade Cleaning Wipes

Total Time: 3 min

Ingredients

- Water – 1 cup
- Distilled white vinegar – 1 cup
- Liquid dish detergent – 3 drops
- Lemon essential oil – 20 drops
- Paper towels or washcloths – 36
- Container

Instructions

1. If using washcloths, cut them into 36 square sizes.

2. Mix all other ingredients in a bowl, then pour over the towels.

3. Shake gently to get the towels well saturated.

4. Use when needed.

Note: do not use on marble, granite or other natural stones.

How to Use Cleaning Wipes

- Use the wipes to clean up messes and spills on your kitchen counters

- Wipe the handle of your cart when shopping

- Clean out your microwave

- Clean up streaks on ovens, dishwaters, and refrigerators

- Make your kitchen sink clean and sparkling

- Clean and disinfect your toilet seats and sinks.

- Eliminate mildew and mold from your bathroom: wipe the affected surfaces with the disinfectant wipes. Leave it to air dry.

- Clean out your car's interiors.

How to Use Wipes to Disinfect Surfaces

1. The first thing to do is use the cleaning wipe or cleaning spray to clean dirty surfaces.

2. Then use the wipe on the surfaces.

3. Wipe the surfaces until it is clearly wet

4. Then allow to air dry.

Chapter 2: How to Make Hand Sanitizer and Home Disinfectant with Essential Oils

Do you know that there are different categories of hand sanitizers? They are generally classified according to the type of active ingredients inside it. The two main categories are Alcohol-Based Sanitizers and Alcohol-Free Hand Sanitizers.

Let us take a look at what defines the categories.

Alcohol-based Sanitizers

As the name suggests, alcohol-based hand sanitizers have alcohol ingredients inside. Generally, these hand sanitizers contain between 60 - 95% isopropanol, ethanol, or n-propanol. The alcohol in those concentrations automatically denaturalizes proteins, making these sanitizers the best at combatting dangerous viruses, and specific microorganisms.

Some alcohol-based sanitizers contain a compound known as glycerol. Glycerol is effective in preventing the skin from being dry, especially after using hand sanitizer.

Natural Alcohol-Free Sanitizers

These hand sanitizers have absolutely no alcohol ingredients. They are generally called disinfectants that have antimicrobial agents and benzalkonium chloride (BAC).

The efficacy of alcohol-free sanitizers is usually based on the ingredients and the mixture content, and that is why they perform less than alcohol-based sanitizers. However, formulas that use BAC have shown to have increased antimicrobial activity after application because it stays longer in hand even after drying. The same cannot be said of alcohol-based sanitizers.

Antiseptic Spray

This simple spray may be used on hands and countertops.

Time: 7 mins.

Yield: 2.5 cups

Ingredients:

2 tbsp. Aloe Vera gel

1 tbsp. Witch Hazel

10 drops Lavender oil

2 tsp. Vitamin E oil

10 drops Frankincense oil

10 drops Tea tree oil

2 cups Water

Directions:

1. Mix all the ingredients together such as witch hazel, aloe Vera gel, vitamin E oil, Lavender oil, tea tree oil and frankincense oil in a bottle.

2. Then add water in it and shake it well.

3. Cover it and let it store for a bit, after a while spray the sanitizer and enjoy the hygiene.

The Natural Spray

This sanitizer spray is made solely from natural ingredients and is alcohol free.

Time: 7 mins.

Yield: 0.5 cups

Ingredients:

2 tbsp. Witch hazel

2 tbsp. Water

1 tbsp. Vegetable glycerin

5 drops Lemongrass essential oil

20 drops Tea tree oil

5 drops Rosemary essential oil

Directions:

1. Get a bottle with the cap and the spray on it.

2. Add water first and then combine all the following ingredients in it such as witch hazel, vegetable glycerin, tea tree oil, lemongrass oil and rosemary oil together.

3. Blend it together. Spritz the spray on your hand for 2-3 times and then rub it together for it to dry.

Ginger Sanitizer Spray

Ginger is great for ridding your body of viruses, and the same goes for this sanitizer.

Time: 5 mins.

Yields: 2.5 cup

Ingredients

2 cups water

5 drops Tea tree oil

5 drops ginger essential oil

½ tbsp. Aloe Vera gel

1 tbsp. Rubbing alcohol

Directions

1. Pour and mix all listed ingredients together in a bowl and stir well.

2. Blend the mixture.

Tarragon Sanitizer Spray

This mixture is simple and will keep you protected.

Time: 5 mins.

Yields: 2.5 cups

Ingredients

2 cups water

5 drops Tea tree oil

5 drops tarragon essential oil

½ tbsp. Aloe Vera gel

1 tbsp. Rubbing alcohol

Directions

1. Pour and mix all listed ingredients together in a bowl and stir well.

2. Blend the mixture.

Cinnamon Sanitizer Spray

Cinnamon essential oil is great for aromatherapy as it smells great and is great for your skin.

Time: 5 mins.

Yields: 2.5 cups

Ingredients

2 cups water

5 drops Tea tree oil

5 drops cinnamon essential oil

½ tbsp. Aloe Vera gel

1 tbsp. Rubbing alcohol

Directions

1. Pour and mix all listed ingredients together in a bowl and stir well.

2. Blend the mixture.

Sandalwood Sanitizer Spray

Sandalwood possesses many virus fighting properties.

Time: 5 mins.

Yields: 2.5 cups

Ingredients

2 cups water

5 drops Tea tree oil

5 drops Sandalwood essential oil

½ tbsp. Aloe Vera gel

1 tbsp. Rubbing alcohol

Directions

1. Pour and mix all listed ingredients together in a bowl and stir well.

2. Blend the mixture well and pure then into any container for future use.

Vetiver Sanitizer Spray

This Vetiver sanitizer is smooth on the skin and leaves your skin moist.

Time: 5 mins.

Yields: 2.5 cups

Ingredients

2 cups water

5 drops Tea tree oil

5 drops vetiver essential oil

½ tbsp. Aloe Vera gel

1 tbsp. Rubbing alcohol

Directions

1. Pour and mix all listed ingredients together in a bowl and stir well.

2. Blend the mixture well and pure then into any container for future use.

Lavender Sanitizer Spray

This lavender sanitizer has a refreshing scent and is good for the skin.

Time: 5 mins.

Yields: 2.5 cups

Ingredients

2 cups water

5 drops Tea tree oil

5 drops lavender essential oil

½ tbsp. Aloe Vera gel

1 tbsp. Rubbing alcohol

Directions

1. Pour and mix all listed ingredients together in a bowl and stir well.

2. Blend the mixture well and pure then into any container for future use.

Lemon Tea Tree Oil Gel Spray

This easy homemade sanitizer makes for a delightful spray that is easy on the skin.

Time: 5 mins.

Yields: 2.5 cups

Ingredients

2 cups water

5 drops Tea tree oil

5 drops lemon essential oil

½ tbsp. Aloe Vera gel

1 tbsp. Rubbing alcohol

Directions

1. Pour and mix all listed ingredients together in a bowl and stir well.

2. Blend the mixture well and pure then into any container for future use.

Anise sanitizer Spray

Anise is an essential oil known to have great anti-bacterial properties.

Time: 5 mins.

Yields: 2.5 cups

Ingredients

2 cups water

5 drops Tea tree oil

5 drops anise essential oil

½ tbsp. Aloe Vera gel

1 tbsp. Rubbing alcohol

Directions

1. Pour and mix all listed ingredients together in a bowl and stir well.

2. Blend the mixture well and pure then into any container for future use.

Cedarwood Sanitizer Spray

This sanitizer is nutrient filled and great for your skin.

Time: 5 mins.

Yields: 2.5 cups

Ingredients

2 cups water

5 drops Tea tree oil

5 drops Cedarwood essential oil

½ tbsp. Aloe Vera gel

1 tbsp. Rubbing alcohol

Directions

1. Pour and mix all listed ingredients together in a bowl and stir well.

2. Blend the mixture well and pure then into any container for future use.

Caraway Sanitizer Spray

This Caraway sanitizer is alcohol-based yet very light on the skin.

Time: 5 mins.

Yields: 2.5 cups

Ingredients

2 cups water

5 drops Tea tree oil

5 drops caraway essential oil

½ tbsp. Aloe Vera gel

1 tbsp. Rubbing alcohol

Directions

1. Pour and mix all listed ingredients together in a bowl and stir well.

2. Blend the mixture well and pure then into any container for future use.

Fennel Sanitizer Spray

Fennel has a unique smell that adds a slightly minty scent to your sanitizer.

Time: 5 mins.

Yields: 2.5 cups

Ingredients

2 cups water

5 drops Tea tree oil

5 drops fennel essential oil

½ tbsp. Aloe Vera gel

1 tbsp. Rubbing alcohol

Lemon Essential Oil Hand Wash

This hand wash can be prepared in as little as 5 minutes and is the perfect travel size portion.

Time: 5 mins.

Yields: 1.5 cups

Ingredients

¾ cup water

¼ cup castile soap

20 drops lemon essential oil

Soap dispenser

Directions

1. Wash and rinse out any oil soap dispenser.

2. Pour ¾ cups of water into the dispenser.

3. Add ¼ cups of castile soap.

4. Add in your lemon oil to your mixture.

5. Place the dispenser lid and shake well.

DIY Liquid Hand Soap Spray

DIY liquid hand wash is simply one of the easiest natural recipes that you can make.

Time: 5 mins.

Yields: 1.5 cups

Ingredients

5-10 drops lavender oil

1 TB olive oil or jojoba oil or sweet almond oil

½ cup distilled water

1/2 cup of castile soap liquid

1 TB vitamin E oil (optional)

15 drops tea tree oil

Directions

1. In a recycled soap dispenser or mason jar, add the water, and then the liquid castle soap, then add the essential oils.

2. Stir the mixture thoroughly to produce a clear solution.

3. Always shake the soap mixture before using it, then apply a small amount on your hand as required.

Rosemary Castor Oil Sanitizer Spray

This mix will blow you away while keeping you protected.

Time: 5 mins.

Yields: 2.5 cups

Ingredients

2 cups water

5 drops castor oil

5 drops rosemary essential oil

½ tbsp. Aloe Vera gel

1 tbsp. Rubbing alcohol

Directions

1. Pour and mix all listed ingredients together in a bowl and stir well.

2. Blend the mixture well and pure then into any container for future use.

Eucalyptus and Bergamot Sanitizer Spray with Vinegar

This simple mix is very effective at ridding viruses.

Time: 7 mins.

Yield: 7 ounces

Ingredients:

2 tbsp. white vinegar

10 tbsp. water

3 – 4 drops bergamot essential oil

3 – 4 drops eucalyptus essential oil

2 tbsp. vodka

Glass measuring cup

Glass spray bottle

Label

Directions:

1. Measure water, vinegar, vodka, and essential oils and pour into the glass measuring cup.

2. Pour into the glass spray bottle. Tighten the spray cap and shake the bottle vigorously until well combined.

3. Label the bottle with name and date.

Grapefruit and Tea Tree Hand Sanitizer with Hydrogen Peroxide

This sanitizer is light, simple and effective.

Time: 7 mins.

Yield: 6 ounces

Ingredients:

2/3 cup rubbing or isopropyl alcohol, more than 60%

½ tbsp. hydrogen peroxide

1 tsp. glycerol

10 drops tea tree essential oil

10 drops grapefruit essential oil

2 tbsp. distilled water

Glass measuring cup

Glass spray bottle

Label

Funnel

Directions:

1. Measure water, alcohol, glycerol, and hydrogen peroxide one at a time and add into the glass spray bottle. Add essential oils.

2. Next, tighten the cap and shake the bottle until well combined.

3. Label the bottle with name and date.

How to use:

Spray all over your hands, including palms, back of the hands, fingers, in between the fingers, nails, and fingertips. Rub into your hands thoroughly. Let it air dry.

Kid-Friendly Hand Sanitizer Spray

This is how to make a kid-safe sanitizer.

Time: 5 mins.

Yield: 2 ounces

Ingredients

½ tsp. Vegetable glycerin

10 drops Spruce essential oil

20 drops Tea tree essential oil

6 drops Lemon essential oil

4 tbsp. 190 proof vodka

Directions

1. Add the essential oils and the glycerin in a 2-ounce spray bottle. Then add the alcohol enough to get the bottle almost full.

2. Cover the lid and shake the bottle thoroughly to mix the ingredients.

3. Shake the bottle each time you want to use it and spray a generous amount in your hand. Rub together, then air dry.

Hand Sanitizer with Aloe Vera Gel

Here we have a sanitizer that is fully natural and healthy.

Time: 5 mins.

Yield: 1.5 cups

Ingredients:

1/3 cup aloe vera gel

2/3 cup Isopropanol

20 drops cinnamon bark oil

20 drops tea tree/peppermint oil

½ tsp glycerin (optional)

Empty, clean spray bottles

Directions:

1. Put all ingredients in a clean pot and stir fully.

2. Now fill the hand disinfectant into a blank spray bottle.

Grapefruit-Aloe Hand Sanitizer Spray

Grapefruit pairs well with Aloe Vera in this simple sanitizer.

Time: 5 mins.

Yield: 1 cup

Ingredients

½ tsp. Vegetable glycerin

¼ cup Aloe vera gel

1 tbsp. Rubbing alcohol

10 drops Tea tree essential oil

10 drops Grapefruit essential oil

Distilled water

Directions

1. Combine the rubbing alcohol, glycerin, and aloe vera gel in a little bowl.

2. Add the tea tree and grapefruit essential oil to the bowl then stir together.

3. Now add the distilled water, little at a time, till you get your wanted consistency.

4. Shift to your bottle or spray.

5. Use as needed.

Safe Sprays for Kids

This herbal hand sanitizer solution does not dry the skin. Actually, it is nourishing because of the addition of aloe vera.

Time: 5 mins.

Yields: 0.5 cup

Ingredients

20 drops Germ Destroyer Essential Oil (This is kid friendly or safe)

1/4 cup aloe Vera gel

Directions

1. Combine your ingredients then place in a silicone tube container.

2. Shift to your bottle or spray.

3. Lastly, use as needed.

Chamomile Oil Spray

The hand sanitizer can be made or produced in the plastic container you plan to use, so you do not have to get a bowl dirty.

Time: 5 mins.

Yields: 1 cup

Ingredients

2 cups water

5 drops Tea tree oil

15 drops Chamomile essential oil

½ tbsp. Aloe Vera gel

1 tbsp. Rubbing alcohol

Directions

1. Pour and mix all listed ingredients together in a bowl and stir well.

2. Blend the mixture well and pure then into any container for future use.

Fir Needle Sanitizer Spray

Use the Fir needle essential cleansing and healing oil in your regular blends and aromatherapy preparations long.

Time: 5 mins.

Yields: 2.5 cups

Ingredients

2 cups water

5 drops Tea tree oil

15 drops Fir needle essential oil

½ tbsp. Aloe Vera gel

1 tbsp. Rubbing alcohol

Directions

1. Pour and mix all listed ingredients together in a bowl and stir well.

2. Blend the mixture well and pure then into any container for future use.

Balsam Fir Sanitizer Spray

Balsam Fir is great for strengthening a healthy respiratory system.

Time: 5 mins.

Yields: 2.5 cups

Ingredients

2 cups water

5 drops Tea tree oil

15 drops Balsam Fir essential oil

½ tbsp. Aloe Vera gel

1 tbsp. Rubbing alcohol

Directions

1. Pour and mix all listed ingredients together in a bowl and stir well.

2. Blend the mixture well and pure then into any container for future use.

Tea Tree Douglas Fir Sanitizer Spray

The properties of both tea tree oil and Douglas fir join forces in this sanitizer mix.

Time: 5 mins.

Yields: 2.5 cups

Ingredients:

2 cups water

5 drops Tea tree oil

15 drops Douglas Fir essential oil

½ tbsp. Aloe Vera gel

1 tbsp. Rubbing alcohol

Directions

1. Pour and mix all listed ingredients together in a bowl and stir well.

2. Blend the mixture well and pure then into any container for future use.

White Fir Sanitizer Spray

White Fir carries a ton of benefits all of which are great for your skin.

Time: 5 mins.

Yields: 2.5 cups

Ingredients

2 cups water

5 drops Tea tree oil

15 drops White Fir essential oil

½ tbsp. Aloe Vera gel

1 tbsp. Rubbing alcohol

Directions

1. Pour and mix all listed ingredients together in a bowl and stir well.

2. Blend the mixture well and pure then into any container for future use.

Peppermint Sanitizer Spray

The peppermint is known as flowers and leaves are harvested to extract the essential oil from them that is great for your skin.

Time: 5 mins.

Yields: 2.5 cups

Ingredients

2 cups water

5 drops Tea tree oil

15 drops Peppermint essential oil

½ tbsp. Aloe Vera gel

1 tbsp. Rubbing alcohol

Directions

1. Pour and mix all listed ingredients together in a bowl and stir well.

2. Blend the mixture well and pure then into any container for future use.

Chapter 3: Sanitizer Recipes

One of my preferred custom-made All-Purpose Cleaners is planned with a couple of basic fixings that I know are successful in cleaning family unit surfaces. Hydrogen Peroxide (3%): This normal medication bureau staple can eliminate microscopic organisms, shape, buildup, and parasite. It is recorded with the Environmental Protection Agency as a sterilizer. It tends to be utilized to sanitize every one of your surfaces in the kitchen and washroom, evacuate recolors, and even to clean mirrors and hardened steel. I like to utilize its full quality since it is as of now weakened (3% hydrogen peroxide, 97% water) when you buy it.

Note: Hydrogen peroxide is delicate to light so it must be kept either in its unique container (with an additional spray spout) or moved to another dark spray bottle.

Essential Oils: Essential oils are the unpredictable oils separated from different pieces of plants.

Notwithstanding their awesome fragrance, certain essential oils are known for their antibacterial, antifungal, clean, and germicidal properties. I love adding essential oils to a DIY cleaner to additionally improve its viability.

Something else? Not a lot. This is the manner by which you keep DIY cleaners extremely basic, modest, and powerful!

Appreciate this recipe.
Natively constructed All Purpose Cleaner: Lavender Mint
Fixings
• opaque spray bottle or the first hydrogen peroxide bottle with included spray spout
• 16 oz. hydrogen peroxide (3%)
• ½ teaspoon lavender essential oil
• ½ teaspoon lemon essential oil

- ⅛ teaspoon peppermint essential oil

Guidelines

Join all fixings in bottle, append spray spout, and shake to consolidate. For best purifying outcomes, spray on surfaces and leave for several minutes before cleaning off.

Hand crafted Sanitizer Spray

This hand-crafted sanitizer spray is the thing that I use for regular cleaning and sanitizing. We have a ton of kid toys, so I keep a major jug on hand. It is normal and safe while as yet working admirably of cleaning toys and considerably more.

Fixings

- 1 cup refined white vinegar
- 1 cup refined water
- 30 drops lavender essential oil

Directions

1. Combine all fixings in a huge spray bottle.
2. Liberally spray toys and permit the blend to sit for 1-2 minutes.
3. Wipe clean with a sodden fabric and permit toys to air dry.

Notes

This strategy works for all toys that can endure being sprayed with water. For electronic toys, I spray a fabric with the sanitizing spray first and afterward wipe toys.

Borax and Castile Soap Cleaner

This hand crafted generally useful cleaner with essential oils is useful for cleaning pretty much everything. We use it a ton in the kitchen, shower, and toilet bowl, and washroom. Despite the fact that it has cleanser in it, you do not have to wash it on most surfaces. The modest quantity of cleanser effectively wipes up and does not leave a film. On glass or extremely sparkling surfaces, give it a flush with a wet material.

Recipes

- 1 tsp washing soda
- 2 tsp Borax
- 2 tsp liquid Castile cleanser

- 15 drops orange essential oil, discretionary
- 5 drops lavender essential oil, discretionary
- 1-quart high temp water

Guidance

I like to blend this up in a quart spray bottle, ideally glass, and save it on hand for ordinary use, as its outstanding amongst other natively constructed characteristic cleaners you can have. You can discover Borax (not the acid) and washing soda in the clothing cleanser segment of most markets. I like to utilize refined water to abstain from deserting water spots.

Generally useful Disinfectant

It is anything but difficult to make your own disinfectant spray with family unit fixings. This disinfectant works superior to fade, without the stress of taking in unsafe synthetic compounds. It is basically a blend of equivalent bits of hydrogen peroxide and vinegar, yet it must be made and utilized quickly since the disinfectant characteristics do not last after some time. My inclination is to keep two spray bottles: one of hydrogen peroxide and one of white vinegar.

Recipe
- 1 part refined white vinegar
- 1 part 3% hydrogen peroxide

I spray the surface with vinegar and afterward peroxide and combine them with a wipe or delicate fabric. Leave them superficially for a couple of moments to do their enchantment.

I utilize this as a custom-made kitchen cleaner to sterilize in the kitchen, washroom, children's toys, and some other surface that I need germ free. Be cautious with textures, however, as hydrogen peroxide has a gentle fading activity and can stain dim materials.

Vinegar Based Homemade Multi-Purpose sanitizing cleaner

I am constantly somewhat careful of vinegar-based cleaners since they can destroy a few completions, so consistently check your cleaning guidelines before utilizing vinegar. On the in addition to side, vinegar is a fantastic degreaser, which makes it the ideal custom-made stove cleaner. We like to utilize this cleaner for oily surfaces, glass, and other sparkling surfaces.

There are such a significant number of employments for vinegar in the home that you ought to consistently keep an enormous jug on hand with your other cleaning supplies, just as in the washroom for cooking. Vinegar is a brilliant device for how to expel rust from hardened steel, just as cleaning the surface with the goal that it glimmers. Make certain to follow the grain of the spotless machine with the goal that you do not start to expose what's underneath.

Recipe
- ½ cup refined white vinegar
- 2 tbsp. baking soda
- 3 drops of tea tree oil
- Distilled water to fill the container

Make this custom-made multipurpose cleaner in a quart spray container and save it on hand for general cleaning undertakings. It will froth a little when you blend it, so leave a little room at the highest point of the jug and include the water gradually. This recipe is even proper for how to clean a treated steel cooler, just as your different hardened steel machines.

Include this vinegar cleaning solution for washroom cleaning and for the kitchen, also. Vinegar is extraordinary to clean cover floors and is the base element for the absolute best custom-made floor cleaner recipes.

Homespun Cleaners That Actually Work well according to experts

The common fixings you need very well might be stowing away in your washroom.

A portion of the things in your storeroom (like baking soda and vinegar) function as viable generally useful cleaners and, far superior, cost by nothing. So, whenever you are gazing intently at a major chaos however, you are out of your preferred cleaning item, do not hurry to the store — attempt one stirring up one of these DIY customs made cleaners instead. These regular items will kick grime to the check and keep your wallet upbeat.

Significant Safety Tip: Never join alkali-based cleaners with chlorine blanch or items containing fade, for example, powdered dishwasher cleanser. The exhaust they will make are incredibly hazardous. Prior to doing any blending, read the item marks first. Continuously mark any jugs of DIY cleaners with all the fixings inside. If you that a youngster or creature gets into it, it is imperative to realize what the blend contains.

Scented All-Purpose Cleaner

What you will require:
•One-part white vinegar
•One-part water
•Lemon skin
•Rosemary sprigs

Consolidate the above fixings together, fill a spray container, shake, and afterward let implant for seven days before utilizing. When done, you can utilize the normal solution to evacuate hard water stains, clean waste jars, wipe away divider smirches, and substantially more. Other than a crisp aroma, the lemon skin may help support cleaning power. Alert: Do not utilize acidic cleaners on rock, as they will draw the stone.

Kitchen hand Cleaner and Deodorizer

What you will require:
•4 tbsps. baking soda
•1-quart warm water

To clean kitchen counters, apparatuses, and within your cooler, all you need is baking soda. It causes an extraordinary to deodorizer and can be utilized to spark tempered steel sinks and machines. To freshen up surfaces, utilize the solution above or pour baking soda directly from the container and into your channel or waste disposal to evacuate scents. To sparkle and expel spots from hardened steel, make a glue of baking soda and water. Apply it with a soggy fabric and rub tenderly toward the metal's grain. Wash and buff dry.

DIY Glass Cleaner

What you will require:

•2 cups water

•1/2 cup white or juice vinegar

•1/4 cup hydrogen peroxide 70% fixation

•Optional 2-3 drops of orange essential oil for smell

Whenever you have to wash your windows and mirrors, join these fixings and pour them in a spray bottle.

Indication: Don't perfect windows on a hot, radiant day, in light of the fact that the solution will dry too rapidly and leave heaps of streaks. Spray the solution first on a paper towel or delicate material first before cleaning, if you are cleaning mirrors.

Hand crafted Brass Cleaner

What you will require:

•White vinegar or lemon juice

•Table salt

To clean non-lacquered bureau pulls, restroom arrangements, and the sky is the limit from there, hose a wipe with vinegar or lemon juice, at that point sprinkle on salt. Daintily rub over surface. Wash completely with water, at that point promptly dry with a clean delicate fabric.

DIY Grease Cleaner

What you will require:

•1/2 cup sudsy smelling salts

Sudsy smelling salts contains cleanser that helps expel extreme grime. Blend 1/2 of a cup with enough water to fill a gallon holder. At that point clean your broiler racks, stove hood, and barbecue by dunking a wipe into the solution and cleaning over the surface before flushing with clear water. You can likewise douse broiler racks and barbecue grinds in the blend straightforwardly, with some additional smelling salts if you that they are especially grimy.

Final Resort Clothing Stain Remover

What you will require:

•1-gallon boiling water

•1 cup powdered dishwasher cleanser

•1 cup standard liquid chlorine blanch, not ultra or concentrate

Treat seriously recolored however launder able white dress by blending the above fixings into a hardened steel, plastic, or finish bowl (not aluminum). Splash article of clothing for 15-20 minutes. In the event that stain is still there, let it douse somewhat more, at that point wash the thing not surprisingly.

Characteristic Marble Cleaner

What you will require:

•2 drops gentle dishwashing liquid

•2 cups warm water

Blend dishwashing cleanser and water whenever you need to clean normal stone ledges. Wipe over marble then flush totally to expel any cleanser buildup. Buff with a delicate fabric; do not let the marble air-dry. Alert: Never use vinegar, lemon, or some other acidic cleaner on marble or rock surfaces; it will gradually erode into the stone.

Chapter 4: How Hand Sanitizer Works

Most sanitizer companies boast about how their products kill 99.9% of germs. But how true is this? Is it a myth or a fact? Well, the key component in most hand sanitizers is alcohol. The alcohol in sanitizers kills harmful bacteria and viruses by splitting their proteins or affecting their metabolism. According to Clinical Microbiology, solutions that contain at least 30% of alcohol can kill some pathogens. The potency of this solution increases with the concentration of alcohol.

For the recipes I am going to teach you, your homemade hand sanitizer should contain more than 60% alcohol to effectively kill most of the germs on your hands.

Hand sanitizers function by removing the external film on your skin.

The effectiveness of your hand sanitizer depends on several factors.

Proper way to use a hand sanitizer

Applying sanitizer your hands seems pretty straightforward — Apply on hands and rub. Still, there is a method for adequate hand sanitizing techniques: Yes, there is a proper way to use a hand sanitizer. You may have been using it wrong. Well, applying your hand sanitizer is not rocket science. Instead, in less than 30 seconds, you can fight off those germs when you apply it correctly. To make things even easier, I have compiled the process into small and easy steps.

Step 1: First, remove all dirt and greasy stains from your hands.

Step 2: Spray or Apply a dime-size amount on the palm of one hand.

Step 3: Stroke your hands together, ensure you cover all the areas on both hands.

Top tip: Pay close attention to areas between your fingers, and around your fingertips and nails.

Step 4: Rub your hands together for at least 30 seconds to allow your hands to absorb the product completely.

Step 5: Allow your hand sanitizer to dry off completely before you touch any substance.

That is it. Whether you are out in the grocery store, using a public restroom, stuck in traffic, or even using the gas pump, you can sanitize your hand correctly with these 5 easy steps.

How effective is your Homemade Sanitizer?

Before you dive into the recipes, there is one aspect many people ignore – The effectiveness of their homemade hand sanitizer. Since you have made the smart plan to produce your hand sanitizer, there are some factors to consider. Firstly, you must measure your ingredients accurately to ensure your sanitizer maintains its effectiveness. Otherwise, your homemade sanitizer may cause more harm than good. Another essential factor you should consider is the percentage of alcohol. On your old sanitizer bottle, the alcohol may be listed as itemized as ethanol, ethyl alcohol, or isopropyl alcohol. Regardless of the type of alcohol and other ingredients, your sanitizer should have an alcohol percentage of at least 60%. If the concentration falls below 60% [alcohol content], the sanitizer also loses its effectiveness in killing germs.

Benefits of having a readily available Homemade Sanitizer

Your homemade hand sanitizer can be an invaluable accessory, especially if you are a mother with kids running about and touching almost everything they see. Unfortunately, most sanitizers contain alcohol, and this can be sensitive to their skin.

Well, making your homemade sanitizers with simple, all-natural ingredients that will not irritate and dry out your skin, is within reach.

With just a few essential oils, you can create your own readily available homemade hand sanitizer.

How to Wash your hands properly

You touch people, your face, office papers, and as you are reading this, maybe you are touching your computer. Regardless of where you touch, germs find their way of accumulating on your hands. Unfortunately, you do not only risk infecting yourself when you touch your eyes, nose, or mouth. You can also spread it to others.

Although it can be far fetching always to keep your hands free of harmful bacteria and viruses, washing your hands is the best bet to keep your hands germ-free.

Washing your hand correctly, does not have to be complicated. I have compiled the technique into 5 easy steps.

Step 1: Switch on your tap and wet your hands (to the wrist). Switch off the tap and rub an adequate amount of soap.

Top tip: The temperature of the water does not matter.

Step 2: Rub your hands together to form a lather. Pay close attention to the backs of your hands, between your fingers, under your nails, and way back up to your wrists.

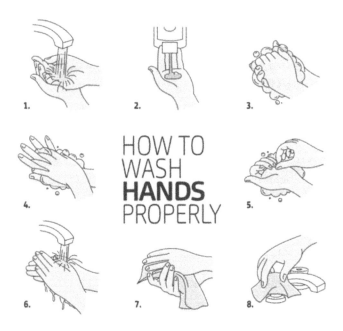

Step 3: Scrub your hands for at least 20 seconds.

Top tip: To make your handwashing process more enjoyable, you can sing a short song to get your timing right.

Step 4: Re-open your tab and rinse your hands thoroughly under clean running water using the same technique.

Step 5: Finally, you can try your hand using a clean paper towel, a hand dryer, or you can allow your hands to air dry.

Homemade Sanitizers

Homemade Sanitizers became even more recognized in 2019 – and appetites for homemade sanitizers do not seem to be slowing down, either. With the high requests for commercial sanitizers, it has become nearly impossible for drug stores and grocery shops to keep up.

Luckily, this is not necessarily bad news. Besides the suffocating medicinal smell of commercial sanitizers, the dry alcohol in them can also irritate the skin.

Homemade sanitizers are milder for sensitive skin, yet strong enough to use after using public toilets.

Making your homemade sanitizer does not have to be expensive or complicated. Instead, to bolster its already impressive advantages, making your sanitizer at home can save you a lot of money and time.

If you are worried about mixing chemicals with chemicals, you probably have the ingredients right in your kitchen cabinet, or worst-case scenario, you may have to visit the local drug store.

The ingredients for your homemade sanitizer are always readily available. As a bonus, with the recipes you are about to learn, you can give your sanitizer the smell of your choice.

Types of Homemade Sanitizers

Hand sanitizers come in various forms. However, regardless of what form of homemade sanitizer you choose to make, as long as its alcohol concentration is 60% and above – You have an effective sanitizer.

You can make your sanitizer as either.

<u>Gels</u>

When compared to other types of DIY Sanitizers, Gel sanitizers are more cost-effective and are very easy to use.

Foams

Foams are also an excellent choice of homemade sanitizers, especially since they adhere to the hands and reduce the limitation of falling on the ground.

Spray

Sprays are effective, but can be uneconomical, especially since particles can deflect into the air and fall onto the floor.

Essential Ingredients for your homemade sanitizer recipes

Just like every great chef has a secret recipe, every homemade sanitizer has its extraordinary ingredient. In this part, you are going to learn about the ingredients you can use for your homemade sanitizer. With these few ingredients, you can unearth and create your custom hand sanitizer. Let us get started!

1) Vinegar

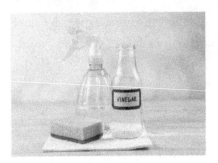

For decades, vinegar has been an invaluable cure for infections, wounds. It also serves as an excellent food preservative and a disinfectant. In recent years, vinegar has proved to be a vital ingredient in sanitizers due to its potent antibacterial property.

It contains antioxidants that repair damaged cells. Vinegar also eliminates harmful bacteria by preventing their multiplication. The environment-friendly ingredient is usually available in drug stores.

Top tip: I recommend you use white vinegar for your homemade sanitizer. If you are not a huge fan of the smell, you can add other sweet-smelling ingredients like lemon or lavender to your sanitizer. Alternatively, you can allow your hands to air dry because the smell of vinegar disperses easily.

2) Aloe Vera

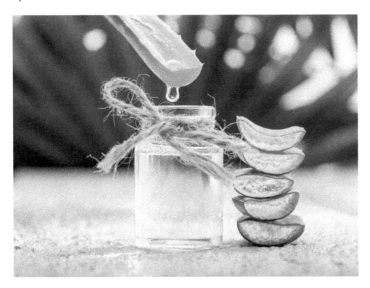

The cell-regenerating Aloe Vera makes a superb addition to our ingredient list and rightly so, this miracle ingredient contains 99% water and about 75 potentially active elements. Aloe's natural healing properties can be credited to its antioxidants, vitamins, enzymes, and antimicrobial properties.

Aloe makes an excellent choice for your homemade sanitizer. Because of its ample water content, Aloe Vera hydrates your hands without leaving the uncomfortable greasy feeling of commercial sanitizers.

3) Alcohol

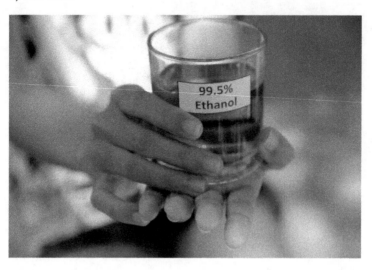

Alcohol is one of the most popular and vital ingredients for your homemade sanitizer. Proof? More than 100 years of practical application. Alcohol works by attacking protein in bacteria, and as a result, kills the cells. However, there is a catch. Using the beer or vodka in your fridge will not be as effective. Your homemade sanitizer needs to have at least 60% alcohol to be effective in fighting germs.

Top tip: I recommend making your sanitizer at least 75% alcohol. If your skin is sensitive and you still find your sanitizer overwhelming, you can add one or two teaspoons of your favorite essential oil to counter this effect.

4) Hydrogen Peroxide

Hydrogen Peroxide makes our ingredient list because of its unbelievable oxidizing power. This robust solution oxidizes when it comes in contact with germs and causes bacteria to decompose.

Although a Hydrogen peroxide-based sanitizer is very easy to use, it can cause a tingling sensation on contact with the skin.

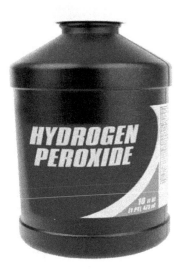

Top tip: If hydrogen peroxide is your preferred ingredient, I recommend you store your hand sanitizer in a dark-colored bottle. Remember to keep it away from sunlight because hydrogen peroxide oxidizes on contact with air.

5) Tea Tree Oil

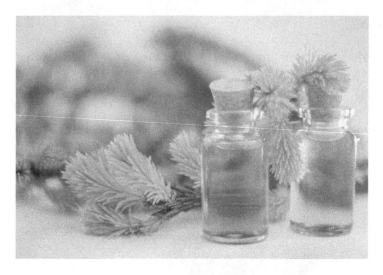

If you are new to the world of essential oils or even a frequent user, then you should know how unique Tea tree oil is, it is a splendid and priceless addition to any collection. Tea tree oil is easily one of our preferred active home ingredients.

Tea tree oil boasts of incredible antiviral, antibacterial, anti-fungal, and anti-inflammatory properties. Since it has potent antiseptic properties, it increases the effectiveness of your homemade hand sanitizer. However, the smell can be pungent.

Top tip: I recommend you properly label your sanitizers because Tea tree oil can be harmful if pregnant women or children ingest it.

Bonus Tip: If your skin is extra sensitive. You can pick one or two essential oils; you do not have to use all of them.

6. Lemon Essential Oil

Lemon essential oil is a natural sweet-smelling antiseptic made from fresh lemons. The essential oil has been around for thousands of years, serving anti-fungal and antibacterial functions.

The lemon essential oil also has brilliant effects on the skin, especially if you are suffering from acne.

Top tip: Although Tea tree oil is a more potent disinfectant, the smell can be stomach-turning. Adding a few drops of Lemon essential oil helps to mask the pungent smell.

7. Winter bloom

The use of Winter bloom as a medical disinfectant has been around for decades. Today, due to its practical applications as an antimicrobial agent, it has become an excellent ingredient for making hand sanitizers. In addition to its already impressive qualities, winter bloom also has a small concentration of Alcohol. You should note that the percentage of Alcohol in winter bloom does not meet the 60% requirement to make an effective sanitizer. Nevertheless, winter bloom makes a potent addition when used with other ingredients. I recommend using winter bloom if your skin is sensitive to Alcohol.

Top tip: Depending on your location, winter bloom is also known as witch hazel.

Other vital ingredients you will need for your homemade sanitizer include.

Bowl: To mix your ingredients

Spoon: To stir your ingredients together.

Funnel: To guide your homemade sanitizer into the labeled bottle.

Whisk: Essential Oils do not mix well with water, and usually, stirring may not be enough. You can use the whisk to whip up your recipe into a homogeneous gel. Plastic bottles: Once you have made the homemade sanitizer of your choice, you will need a safe place to keep it in. I recommend using a transparent bottle with a flip top. The flip-top makes squeezing out your hand sanitizer almost effortless. Gloves: You are creating a unique homemade sanitizer to protect yourself from germs, so it is only logical you stay safe when mixing ingredients. Wearing gloves prevents burns and injuries that could result from spills directly on your hand.

Chapter 5: The Differences Between Cleaning, Disinfecting, and Sanitizing

While we are aiming to achieve cleanliness in our household, it is important to know the differences of the terms in order to apply them appropriately and avoid causing potential problems.

Tidying up the house or any living space is a conventional term that implies various things to various individuals. Your meaning of tidying up to your youngster may mean getting dispersed toys. Tidying up the kitchen can mean simply washing the dishes and taking care of extras. Yet, there are particular meanings of cleaning, purifying, and sanitizing surfaces in homes, schools, and open spots. These definitions are set by the Centers for Disease Control and Prevention (CDC) to characterize the degree of microbial defilement left on a surface after treatment.

For a mortgage holder, the terms will assist you with perusing item names and decide whether the items you are utilizing are giving the best possible degree of sanitation required in the event that somebody in your house is sick or has an undermined invulnerable framework.

Cleaning

Cleaning is the way toward evacuating noticeable flotsam and jetsam, earth, and dust and sorting out a space. Cleaning a surface uses cleanser or cleanser and, as a rule, water to evacuate soil and germs through concoction (cleaner), mechanical (scouring), and warm (water temperature) activity.

Cleaning could possibly eliminate microscopic organisms and germs, yet it will weaken their numbers and help in bringing down the danger of spreading irresistible microorganisms.

Disinfecting

At the point when an item professes to sterilize a surface, it is promising to make the surface liberated from germs that could be hurtful to your wellbeing as indicated by general wellbeing gauges or necessities. Disinfecting decreases, not murders, the number and development of microscopic organisms, infections, and growths.

Cleaning is especially significant in nourishment planning zones where germs and organisms can cause nourishment borne diseases. Synthetic concoctions may not be required on the grounds that outrageous warmth—at any rate 170 degrees F—in a dishwasher or by utilizing a steam cleaner can eliminate microscopic organisms.

Sanitizing

The demonstration of cleaning murders minuscule creatures (germs, infections, parasites) on surfaces. Sanitization is typically accomplished by utilizing EPA-affirmed synthetic compounds that execute the living beings and keep them from spreading. Things can likewise be sterilized utilizing UV-C germicidal short frequency, bright light that breaks separated the DNA of microscopic organisms and germs leaving them unfit to hurt or recreate. This is a similar UV-C light innovation utilized in emergency clinic careful suites to help in murdering super-bugs.

Sanitizing does not really expel obvious soil and flotsam and jetsam from a surface and is substantially more successful if fundamental cleaning is done first.

Cleaning ought to be a normal procedure that happens on a day by day, week by week, month to month, and regular premise. Essential housekeeping looks after request, lessens the development of conceivably unsafe life forms, helps monitor bothers, and ensures the speculation you have made in your home and effects.

Sterilization is significant for wellbeing and cleanliness and is especially significant on shared surfaces like ledges, door handles, light switches, touchpads, and any surface that interacts with body liquids. Cleaning bed materials and underpants is considerably more significant than sterilizing dress shirts and slacks.

Moreover, cleaning ought to consistently be done when somebody in the family unit is sick or in the event that somebody has an undermined resistant framework. Adhering to name guidelines and utilizing disinfectants effectively is imperative to executing microorganisms. On the off chance that the item is not utilized accurately, the procedure just offers an incorrect feeling that all is well with the world.

Food Sanitation

All things that come into contact with nourishment must be viably cleaned and sterilized. This is a 4-stage process that expels nourishment squander, earth, oil and crushes nourishment borne ailment pathogens.

The Code does not determine which strategies must be utilized to guarantee the premises and gear are kept in a perfect and sterile condition. Nourishment organizations may utilize a blend of methodology and techniques to meet Code's necessities.

1. Planning

1. Evacuate free earth and nourishment particles.

2. Flush with warm, consumable water.

2. Cleaning

1. Wash with boiling water (60 °C) and cleanser.

2. Flush with clean consumable water.

3. Sterilizing (microorganisms executing stage)

1. Treat with extremely hot, spotless, consumable water (75 °C) for at any rate 2 minutes.

2. Apply sanitizer as coordinated on the mark.

4. Air drying

Leave seats, counters and hardware to air dry. The most sterile approach to dry hardware is in a depleting rack.

After calamities, some nourishment and drink things are risky and must be tossed out. Yet, unharmed, financially arranged nourishment taking all things together metal jars can be made safe. Evacuate the names, altogether wash, flush, and clean the holders with a disinfecting arrangement of one cup of blanch and five gallons of water. Re-mark and incorporate the lapse date.

Enjoying this book?

Please leave a review because we would love to hear your feedback, opinions and advice to create better products and services for you! Thank you for your support. You are greatly appreciated!"

Chapter 6: Hand Sanitizer and Anti-Bacterial Wipes

Use these wipes after visiting the store, touching a shopping cart, or when using public restrooms.

Yield: 30

Total Time: 10mins

Ingredients:

- 1¼ cups rubbing alcohol
- 1 tbsp hydrogen peroxide
- 1 tsp glycerin
- ¼ cup distilled water

Special equipment:

Non-reactive bowl

30 paper towels cut in half

Airtight container with lid

Directions:

1. In a bowl, whisk the rubbing alcohol with the hydrogen peroxide, glycerin, and distilled water.

2. Fold neatly and stack the paper towels in your chosen container.

3. Pour the rubbing alcohol mixture over the paper towels.

4. Put the lid on the container and shake thoroughly to ensure that all the towels are soaked evenly and entirely.

5. To use: Shake well and wring the wipe out before use.

6. Wipe all over your hands for 20-30 seconds, and air dry.

Basic Hand Sanitizing Wipes

These DIY hand wipes are ideal when soap and hot water are not readily available.

Yield: 15

Total Time: 20mins

Ingredients:

¼ cup hot water

2 tbsp pure aloe vera gel

1½ cups 99% rubbing alcohol

Special equipment:

15-20 kitchen paper towels or small even-size clean rags

Baby wipes container or coffee canister

Mixing bowl

Spoon

Directions:

1. It is important to ensure that all your special equipment is sanitized. You can do this using boiling water. Dry all equipment thoroughly.

1. Fold or roll the towels or rags into your chosen container.

2. In a bowl, combine the hot water with the aloe vera gel and rubbing alcohol. Stir with a spoon to incorporate entirely.

3. Pour the mixture over the towels and into your chosen container, until saturated.

7. To use: Shake well and wring the wipe out before use.

8. Wipe all over your hands for 20-30 seconds, and air dry.

Disinfectant Hand Wipes

Make DIY hand sanitizer wipes in minutes. These portable wipes are convenient and ideal for those times when hand washing is not an option.

Yield: 6

Total Time: 10mins

Ingredients:

⅓ cup 91% rubbing alcohol

1 tbsp aloe vera gel

10 drops vitamin E oil

10 drops lavender essential oil

5 drops tea tree essential oil

Special equipment:

10 small-size kitchen paper towels

Baby wipe container or coffee canister

Mixing cup with a spout

Spoon

Directions:

1. It is important to ensure that all your special equipment is sanitized. You can do this using boiling water. Dry all equipment thoroughly.

2. Fold the paper towels and add them to your chosen container.

3. In a bowl, combine the rubbing alcohol with the aloe vera get until incorporated.

4. Next, add the vitamin E oil, lavender essential oil, and tea tree essential oil.

5. Pour the mixture over the wipes to soak entirely.

6. Replace the lid and use it as needed.

7. To use: Shake well and wring the wipe out before use.

8. Wipe all over your hands for 20-30 seconds, and air dry.

Grapefruit, Tea Tree and Bergamot Wipes

Eco-friendly and non-toxic, these fragrant wipes work well in just 20 seconds. What is more, no hot water or hand towels needed.

Yield: 20

Total Time: 35mins

Ingredients:

1 cup 99% rubbing alcohol

1 tbsp hydrogen peroxide

1 tsp glycerin

¼ cup distilled water

20 drops grapefruit essential oil

10 drops tea tree essential oil

10 drops bergamot essential oil

2½-3 tbsp castile soap

Special equipment:

Mason jar with lid

1 piece of white cotton cloths (cut into even-size squares)

Label

Directions:

1. In a bowl, whisk the rubbing alcohol with the hydrogen peroxide, glycerin, and distilled water.

2. Pour the rubbing alcohol into the jar.

3. Next, add the grapefruit, tea tree, and bergamot essential oils. Shake liberally to incorporate.

4. Add the castile soap, gently swirling it into the mixture, to combine. Do not shake as it will cause the soap to create suds.

5. Roll the cloth squares all over in the mixture and add them to the jar.

6. Seal with a lid and swirl gently to saturate.

7. To use: Shake well and wring the wipe out before use.

8. Wipe all over your hands for 20-30 seconds, and air dry.

Herbal Anti-Bacterial Hand Wipes

You will love the smell of these handy virus-fighting wipes. They will leave your hands feeling not only satisfyingly clean but also fragrant.

Yield: 1 (8 ounces) jar

Total Time: 50mins

Ingredients:

¼ cup 99% isopropyl alcohol

1 tsp tea tree essential oil

1 tsp lavender essential oil

1 tsp eucalyptus essential oil

½ tsp clove essential oil

½ tsp rosemary essential oil

Special equipment:

15 heavy-duty paper towels (separated on perforations and cut into quarters)

1 (8 ounces) jar

Mixing cup with a spout

Directions:

1. It is important to ensure that all your special equipment is sanitized. You can do this using boiling water. Dry all equipment thoroughly.

2. Roll each paper towel up into a single roll, taking care that you add the new towel under the flap of the towel that went before it. This method will make it easier to take the towels out of the container.

3. Continue with this process until all of the towels are fitted snugly into your jar.

4. In the mixing cup, stir together the alcohol and tea tree, lavender, eucalyptus, clove, and rosemary essential oils. Pour the mixture into the jar.

5. Seal with the lid and set aside undisturbed for 15-30 minutes to allow the towels to absorb the liquid.

6. When the towels are uniformly damp, pour away any excess liquid in the jar.

7. To use: Shake well and wring the wipe out before use.

8. Wipe all over your hands for 20-30 seconds, and air dry.

Lavender and Lemon Antibacterial Wipes

Keep these wipes in the glove box of your car and have one at the ready when you are next on the move.

Yield: 48

Total Time: 45mins

Ingredients:

1½ cups rubbing alcohol

1 tbsp coconut oil (melted)

3 drops lemon essential oil

3 drops lavender essential oil

Special equipment:

48 baby wipes or halved paper towels

Baby wipe container or coffee canister

Bowl

Small pan

Directions:

1. It is important to ensure that all your special equipment is sanitized. You can do this using boiling water. Dry all equipment thoroughly.

2. Fold the baby wipes or napkins and stack them in your chosen container.

3. In a bowl, stir together the rubbing alcohol and melted coconut oil until blended. Stir in the lemon and lavender essential oils.

4. Pour the mixture evenly over the wipes and allow it to saturate into the wipes entirely.

5. Seal with the lid and set aside undisturbed for 15-30 minutes. The dry towels will pick up any excess moisture.

6. When the towels are uniformly damp, pour away any excess liquid in the jar.

7. To use: Shake well and wring the wipe out before use.

8. Wipe all over your hands for 20-30 seconds, and air dry.

9. When the wipes are evenly saturated, pour off the excess liquid.

Natural Hand Sanitizing Wipes

Hand sanitizing wipes are the perfect way to use up those leftover coffee canisters.

Yield: 15-20

Total Time: 45mins

Ingredients:

⅓ cup water

8 ounces 91% rubbing alcohol

3 drops tea tree essential oil

3 drops lavender essential oil

3 drops peppermint essential oil

2 tbsp castile soap

Special equipment:

15 paper towels or clean, even-size cloths

Tupperware container or coffee canister

Directions:

1. It is important to ensure that all your special equipment is sanitized. You can do this using boiling water. Dry all equipment thoroughly.

2. Fold the paper towels of clothes and stack them in your chosen container. If you are using a cylindrical container, roll rather than folding.

3. In a bowl, combine the water with the rubbing alcohol, tea tree, lavender, and peppermint essential oil. Stir to combine and add the soap, stirring to blend.

4. Pour the mixture evenly over the wipes and allow it to saturate into the wipes entirely.

5. Seal with the lid and set aside undisturbed for 15-30 minutes. The dry towels will pick up any excess moisture.

6. When the wipes are uniformly damp, pour away any excess liquid in the jar.

7. To use: Shake well and wring the wipe out before use.

8. Wipe all over your hands for 20-30 seconds, and air dry.

9. When the wipes are evenly saturated, pour off the excess liquid.

No More Germs Hand Sanitizing Wipes

Protect your family, banish bacteria, and wave goodbye to germs with these virus-fighting hand wipes.

Yield: 30-40

Total Time: 25mins

Ingredients:

¼ cup hot water

2 tbsp pure aloe vera gel

1½ cups 99% rubbing alcohol

5 drops wild orange essential oil

5 drops clove essential oil

5 drops cinnamon essential oil

3 drops eucalyptus essential oil

Special equipment:

Dry baby wipes

Baby wipe container

Non-reactive bowl

Metal spoon

Directions:

1. It is important to ensure that all your special equipment is sanitized. You can do this using boiling water. Dry all equipment thoroughly.

2. In a bowl, combine the hot water with the aloe vera gel.

3. Add the rubbing alcohol, stirring to combine.

4. A few drops at a time, add the essential oils (wild orange, clove, cinnamon, and eucalyptus) and mix thoroughly.

5. Fold and stack he dry baby wipes in your chosen container.

6. Pour the mixture over the baby wipes and cover with the lid. Shake the container gently and allow the wipes to absorb the liquid for 10-15 minutes.

7. To use: Shake well and wring the wipe out before use.

8. Wipe all over your hands for 20-30 seconds, and air dry.

Quick Wipes

If you do not have any extra ingredients but need to make a batch of hand wipes, quickly and inexpensively, then look no further than this simple recipe using just three ingredients.

Yield: 48

Total Time: 25mins

Ingredients:

2 cups of warm water

1 cup rubbing alcohol

1 tbsp liquid hand soap

Special equipment:

45-50 kitchen paper towels or small even-size clean rags

Tupperware container

Mixing bowl

Spoon

Directions:

1. It is important to ensure that all your special equipment is sanitized. You can do this using boiling water. Dry all equipment thoroughly.

2. Fold or roll the towels or rags into your chosen container.

3. In a bowl, combine the warm water with rubbing alcohol and liquid hand soap. Stir with a spoon to incorporate entirely.

4. Pour the mixture over the towels and into your chosen container, until saturated.

5. To use: Shake well and wring the wipe out before use.

6. Wipe all over your hands for 20-30 seconds, and air dry.

Tea Tree and Geranium Soothing Wipes

Tea tree and geranium essential oils come together to create a great anti-bacterial, virus-fighting wipe. Both are known for their antiseptic and soothing qualities.

Yield: 48

Total Time: 45mins

Ingredients:

1½ cups rubbing alcohol

1 tbsp almond oil (melted)

3 drops tea tree essential oil

3 drops geranium essential oil

Special equipment:

48 baby wipes or halved paper towels

Baby wipe container or coffee canister

Small pan

Directions:

1. It is important to ensure that all your special equipment is sanitized. You can do this using boiling water. Dry all equipment thoroughly.

2. Fold the baby wipes or napkins and stack them in your chosen container.

3. In a bowl, stir together the rubbing alcohol and melted almond oil until blended. A few drops at a time, add the tea tree and geranium essential oils.

4. Pour the mixture evenly over the wipes and allow it to saturate into the wipes entirely.

5. Seal with the lid and set aside undisturbed for 15-30 minutes. The dry towels will pick up any excess moisture.

6. When the towels are uniformly damp, pour away any excess liquid in the jar.

7. To use: Shake well and wring the wipe out before use.

8. Wipe all over your hands for 20-30 seconds, and air dry.

9. When the wipes are evenly saturated, pour off the excess liquid.

Chapter 7: Homemade Anti-Viral Room Sprays & Air Freshener Recipes

Alcohol-Free Sanitizer with Sage and Tea Tree Oil

**Note: Use this Sage and Tea Tree Sanitizer to keep your hands free of viruses and bacteria.

Time: 7 mins.

Yield: 2 ounces

INGREDIENTS

4 tbsp. alcohol-free witch hazel

10 drops tea tree essential oil

10 drops sage essential oil

5 – 6 drops vitamin E oil

2 ounces glass spray bottle

Small funnel

DIRECTIONS

Add witch hazel into the spray bottle using the funnel. Add essential oils and vitamin E oil.

Tighten the spray cap and shake the bottle until well combined.

Label the bottle with name and date.

Eucalyptus and Bergamot Sanitizer Spray with Vinegar

**Note: This simple mix is very effective at ridding viruses.

Time: 7 mins.

Yield: 7 ounces

INGREDIENTS

2 tbsp. white vinegar

10 tbsp. water

3 – 4 drops bergamot essential oil

3 – 4 drops eucalyptus essential oil

2 tbsp. vodka

Glass measuring cup

Glass spray bottle

Label

DIRECTIONS

Measure water, vinegar, vodka, and essential oils and pour into the glass measuring cup.

Pour into the glass spray bottle. Tighten the spray cap and shake the bottle vigorously until well combined.

Label the bottle with name and date.

Grapefruit and Tea Tree Hand Sanitizer with Hydrogen Peroxide

**Note: This sanitizer is light, simple and effective.

Time: 7 mins.

Yield: 6 ounces

INGREDIENTS

2/3 cup rubbing or isopropyl alcohol, more than 60%

½ tbsp. hydrogen peroxide

1 tsp. glycerol

10 drops tea tree essential oil

10 drops grapefruit essential oil

2 tbsp. distilled water

Glass measuring cup

Glass spray bottle

Label

Funnel

DIRECTIONS

Measure water, alcohol, glycerol, and hydrogen peroxide one at a time and add into the glass spray bottle. Add essential oils.

Then, tighten the cap and shake the bottle until well combined.

Label the bottle with name and date.

How to use:

Spray all over your hands, including palms, back of the hands, fingers, in between the fingers, nails, and fingertips. Rub into your hands thoroughly. Let it air dry.

Kid-Friendly Hand Sanitizer Spray

**Note: This is how to make a kid-safe sanitizer.

Time: 5 mins.

Yield: 2 ounces

INGREDIENTS

½ tsp. Vegetable glycerin

10 drops Spruce essential oil

20 drops Tea tree essential oil

6 drops Lemon essential oil

4 tbsp. 190 proof vodka

DIRECTIONS

Add the essential oils and the glycerin in a 2-ounce spray bottle. Then add the alcohol enough to get the bottle almost full.

Cover the lid and shake the bottle thoroughly to mix the ingredients.

Shake the bottle each time you want to use it and spray a generous amount in your hand. Rub together, then air dry.

Hand Sanitizer with Aloe Vera Gel

**Note: Here we have a sanitizer that is fully natural and healthy.

Time: 5 mins.

Yield: 1.5 cups

INGREDIENTS

1/3 cup aloe vera gel

2/3 cup Isopropanol

20 drops cinnamon bark oil

20 drops tea tree/peppermint oil

½ tsp glycerin (optional)

Empty, clean spray bottles

DIRECTIONS

Put all ingredients in a clean pot and stir fully.

Now fill the hand disinfectant into a blank spray bottle.

Grapefruit-Aloe Hand Sanitizer Spray

**Note: Grapefruit pairs well with Aloe Vera in this simple sanitizer.

Time: 5 mins.

Yield: 1 cup

INGREDIENTS

½ tsp. Vegetable glycerin

¼ cup Aloe vera gel

1 tbsp. Rubbing alcohol

10 drops Tea tree essential oil

10 drops Grapefruit essential oil

Distilled water

DIRECTIONS

Combine the rubbing alcohol, glycerin, and aloe vera gel in a little bowl.

Add the tea tree and grapefruit essential oil to the bowl then stir together.

Now add the distilled water, little at a time, till you get your wanted consistency.

Shift to your bottle or spray.

Use as needed.

Safe Sprays for Kids

**Note: This herbal hand sanitizer solution does not dry the skin. Actually, it is nourishing because of the addition of aloe vera.

Time: 5 mins.

Yields: 0.5 cup

INGREDIENTS

20 drops Germ Destroyer Essential Oil (This is kid friendly or safe)

1/4 cup aloe Vera gel

DIRECTIONS

Combine your ingredients then place in a silicone tube container.

Shift to your bottle or spray.

Lastly, use as needed.

Chamomile Oil Spray

**Note: The hand sanitizer can be made or produced in the plastic container you plan to use, so you do not have to get a bowl dirty.

Time: 5 mins.

Yields: 1 cup

INGREDIENTS

2 cups water

5 drops Tea tree oil

15 drops Chamomile essential oil

½ tbsp. Aloe Vera gel

1 tbsp. Rubbing alcohol

DIRECTIONS

Pour and mix all listed ingredients together in a bowl and stir well.

Blend the mixture well and pure then into any container for future use.

Fir Needle Sanitizer Spray

**Note: Use the Fir needle essential cleansing and healing oil in your regular blends and aromatherapy preparations long.

Time: 5 mins.

Yields: 2.5 cups

INGREDIENTS

2 cups water

5 drops Tea tree oil

15 drops Fir needle essential oil

½ tbsp. Aloe Vera gel

1 tbsp. Rubbing alcohol

DIRECTIONS

Pour and mix all listed ingredients together in a bowl and stir well.

Blend the mixture well and pure then into any container for future use.

Balsam Fir Sanitizer Spray

**Note: Balsam Fir is great for strengthening a healthy respiratory system.

Time: 5 mins.

Yields: 2.5 cups

INGREDIENTS

2 cups water

5 drops Tea tree oil

15 drops Balsam Fir essential oil

½ tbsp. Aloe Vera gel

1 tbsp. Rubbing alcohol

DIRECTIONS

Pour and mix all listed ingredients together in a bowl and stir well.

Blend the mixture well and pure then into any container for future use.

Tea Tree Douglas Fir Sanitizer Spray

**Note: The properties of both tea tree oil and Douglas fir join forces in this sanitizer mix.

Time: 5 mins.

Yields: 2.5 cups

INGREDIENTS

2 cups water

5 drops Tea tree oil

15 drops Douglas Fir essential oil

½ tbsp. Aloe Vera gel

1 tbsp. Rubbing alcohol

DIRECTIONS

Pour and mix all listed ingredients together in a bowl and stir well.

Blend the mixture well and pure then into any container for future use.

White Fir Sanitizer Spray

**Note: White Fir carries a ton of benefits all of which are great for your skin.

Time: 5 mins.

Yields: 2.5 cups

INGREDIENTS

2 cups water

5 drops Tea tree oil

15 drops White Fir essential oil

½ tbsp. Aloe Vera gel

1 tbsp. Rubbing alcohol

DIRECTIONS

Pour and mix all listed ingredients together in a bowl and stir well.

Blend the mixture well and pure then into any container for future use.

Peppermint Sanitizer Spray

**Note: The peppermint is known as flowers and leaves are harvested to extract the essential oil from them that is great for your skin.

Time: 5 mins.

Yields: 2.5 cups

INGREDIENTS

2 cups water

5 drops Tea tree oil

15 drops Peppermint essential oil

½ tbsp. Aloe Vera gel

1 tbsp. Rubbing alcohol

DIRECTIONS

Pour and mix all listed ingredients together in a bowl and stir well.

Blend the mixture well and pure then into any container for future use.

Vanilla Sanitizer Spray

**Note: Vanilla Essential oil makes for a nice smelling yet strong sanitizer.

Time: 5 mins.

Yields: 2.5 cups

INGREDIENTS

2 cups water

5 drops Tea tree oil

15 drops Vanilla essential oil

½ tbsp. Aloe Vera gel

1 tbsp. Rubbing alcohol

DIRECTIONS

Pour and mix all listed ingredients together in a bowl and stir well.

Blend the mixture well and pure then into any container for future use.

Cardamom Sanitizer Spray

**Note: As a well-known essential oil, black cardamom is potent as an antioxidant.

Time: 5 mins.

Yields: 2.5 cups

INGREDIENTS

2 cups water

5 drops Tea tree oil

15 drops Cardamom essential oil

½ tbsp. Aloe Vera gel

1 tbsp. Rubbing alcohol

1 oz. glass spray bottle

DIRECTIONS

Pour and mix all listed ingredients together in a bowl and stir well.

Blend the mixture well and pure then into any container for future use.

Eucalyptus Sanitizer Spray

**Note: Eucalyptus has a ton of anti-bacteria properties, making it perfect for use in homemade cleaning and sanitizer.

Time: 5 mins.

Yields: 2.5 cups

INGREDIENTS

2 cups water

5 drops Tea tree oil

15 drops eucalyptus essential oil

½ tbsp. Aloe Vera gel

1 tbsp. Rubbing alcohol

DIRECTIONS

Pour and mix all listed ingredients together in a bowl and stir well.

Blend the mixture well and pure then into any container for future use.

Lemon Oil Gel Spray

**Note: The use of lemon leaves a refreshing feeling to the users.

Time: 5 mins.

Yields: 2.5 cups

INGREDIENTS

2 cups water

5 drops Tea tree oil

5 drops lemon essential oil

½ tbsp. Aloe Vera gel

1 tbsp. Rubbing alcohol

DIRECTIONS

Pour and mix all listed ingredients together in a bowl and stir well.

Blend the mixture well and pure then into any container for future use.

Rosemary Sanitizer Spray

**Note: This Rosemary sanitizer is both healthy and effective.

Time: 5 mins.

Yields: 2.5 cups

INGREDIENTS

2 cups water

5 drops Tea tree oil

5 drops rosemary essential oil

½ tbsp. Aloe Vera gel

1 tbsp. Rubbing alcohol

DIRECTIONS

Pour and mix all listed ingredients together in a bowl and stir well.

Blend the mixture well and pure then into any container for future use.

Clove Tea Tree Sanitizer Spray

**Note: This Clove Tea Tree Sanitizer is easy to make and is full of anti-bacterial properties.

Time: 5 mins.

Yields: 2.5 cups

INGREDIENTS

2 cups water

5 drops Tea tree oil

5 drops Clove essential oil

½ tbsp. Aloe Vera gel

1 tbsp. Rubbing alcohol

DIRECTIONS

Pour and mix all listed ingredients together in a bowl and stir well.

Blend the mixture well and pure then into any container for future use.

Frankincense Sanitizer Spray

**Note: This sanitizer spray kills bacteria while smelling great.

Time: 5 mins.

Yields: 2.5 cups

INGREDIENTS

2 cups water

5 drops Tea tree oil

5 drops frankincense essential oil

½ tbsp. Aloe Vera gel

1 tbsp. Rubbing alcohol

DIRECTIONS

Pour and mix all listed ingredients together in a bowl and stir well.

Blend the mixture well and pure then into any container for future use.

Sandalwood Sanitizer Spray

**Note: Sandalwood possesses many virus fighting properties.

Time: 5 mins.

Yields: 2.5 cups

INGREDIENTS

2 cups water

5 drops Tea tree oil

5 drops Sandalwood essential oil

½ tbsp. Aloe Vera gel

1 tbsp. Rubbing alcohol

DIRECTIONS

Pour and mix all listed ingredients together in a bowl and stir well.

Blend the mixture well and pure then into any container for future use.

Vetiver Sanitizer Spray

**Note: This Vetiver sanitizer is smooth on the skin and leaves your skin moist.

Time: 5 mins.

Yields: 2.5 cups

INGREDIENTS

2 cups water

5 drops Tea tree oil

5 drops vetiver essential oil

½ tbsp. Aloe Vera gel

1 tbsp. Rubbing alcohol

DIRECTIONS

Pour and mix all listed ingredients together in a bowl and stir well.

Blend the mixture well and pure then into any container for future use.

Chapter 8: Rubbing Alcohol Recipes

Alcohol-based sanitizers

Most sanitizers used in the hospitals are alcohol-based. They serve as very effective alternatives to antiseptic soaps. Alcohol hand rubs used in the hospital serve two important functions: surgical hand disinfection or hygienic hand rubbing. Alcohol sanitizers are more tolerant on the skin compared to antiseptic soaps. The microbiological effects of alcohol-based sanitizers are more effective as compared to antiseptic soap.

Alcohol-free sanitizers

Some manufacturers produce sanitizers using a wide range of ingredients other than alcohol. Examples of such ingredients include benzalkonium chloride, povidone-iodine, or triclosan.

Alcohol-free sanitizers are effective while still on the skin. However, it is an irony that the sanitizer itself may be contaminated due to the absence of alcohol – which in most cases serves as an in-solution preservative.

How Safe is a hand sanitizer?

It is much better to follow the directions and take every precautionary measure to protect us than not following at all. A little effort can save you from getting infected.

You should know that if you are using a hand sanitizer, it may not work perfectly if your hands are greasy or visibly dirty. Works like gardening, playing outside, or preparing food, can leave your hands greasy or dirty. In that case, you should wash your hands with soap and water for the recommended duration.

Health Benefits of Sanitizers

The health benefits of hand sanitizers are indeed not farfetched. Hand sanitizers serve as a part of the ways to keep us safe in times of disease outbreaks. We might not categorically refer to these sanitizers as hand sanitizers, but they served the purposes that hand sanitizers serve nowadays.

Hand sanitizers also help in ensuring that our hands are kept clean for eating and other actions that require us to take our hands to our mouths. They relegate the possibility of taking in germs via the hands and mouth.

In the medical setting, they also help to keep patients and doctors alike, safe and protected.

The list is endless, and if you are one who over time has doubted the credibility of hand sanitizers, then I think you should rethink this. Remember, sanitizers are not a replacement for soap and water.

Note: Sanitizers are most effective when they contain alcohol (at least 60 percent). Also, for maximum function, a large quantity should be applied to the hands and rubbed thoroughly, up to the elbows, for some time. I do not think conservatism is an option in the use of hand sanitizers. Most importantly, make use of sanitizers that you like and ones that have fragrances that go down well with you.

Hand-Sanitizers vs. Hand-wash

If you have been wondering if there's an actual difference between these two liquids, the answer is yes. Hand sanitizers and hand-wash liquids have gained popularity in the past 1 or 2 decades but they serve slightly different purposes for every user.

While a hand-sanitizer is an alcohol-based liquid or gel that helps to lower the number of microorganisms on the hands, a hand-washing liquid is essentially soap in liquid form and you'll need to use water along with it to wash your hands.

Hand-washes are often classified as detergents and have since become permanent fixtures in the kitchen and bathrooms of almost every household within the country and beyond. Sometimes, hand-wash liquids contain antibacterial agents that help to kill pathogenic organisms that are present on the hands. Some hand-wash liquids are also classified as "for children" and for these, the concentration of chemicals is slightly adjusted so that it does not affect their delicate skin.

These liquid soaps, as they are often called, come in various forms, fragrances, and sizes and you can always pick the kind that suits you most. One of the major differences that jump out to any observer of the way hand sanitizers and hand-washes are used is that hand-washes foam when they are being used while sanitizers do not.

When you rub a sanitizer on your hands, it feels like you have just wet your hands with some water but after about 20-30 seconds, it evaporates, leaving your hand clear as though you hadn't applied anything on it. When you're washing your hands, you get to spend a longer amount of time to achieve clean hands and if you're using a hand-wash, you'd need to run your hands through water while rubbing your palms together, before you can get rid of the hand-washing liquid along with the germs that are on your hands.

Making liquid soap at home can be a lot simpler than making a hand-sanitizer and this is because you can make liquid soap out of the leftover bar of soap that you have in your bathroom or kitchen while you'd have to make some unique purchases to whip up a homemade hand sanitizer.

In their rights, hand sanitizers and hand-wash liquids serve a common purpose which is to clear the hands of germs and microorganisms that can cause infections in the body. The hand sanitizer can be described as a more expedient resource when you cannot readily get water to wash your hands with but, liquid soap (or any other kind of soap) is just as important when your hands are visibly greasy or dirty.

When you combine the two by washing your hands with soap and water first and then applying a hand sanitizer, it brings about some rather powerful effects and especially if you're one to get your hands dirty in your place of work, at home or in school.

Precautions while using alcohol-based sanitizers

Cleaning Effectiveness

The first thing you should know is that applying hand sanitizers is not an alternative to washing your hands. It is an element that eradicates bacteria on the hand when applied. However, it does not remove dirt on the palms and wrist, and it attacks germs and bacteria. Medical facilities and hospital staffs utilize hand sanitizer but still need to wash the hands with water and soap for the total cleanliness of the hand. Also, you will find some sanitizer without alcoholic content, and they are less effective in the face of germs and different types of bacteria, so it is advisable to use soap and water in such cases.

Endocrine system interference

Some sanitizers contain triclosan, and it is a component that kills every type of bacteria on the hand, including the good and beneficial bacteria. It contains chemicals that function as endocrine disruptors, which can cause early puberty. It is an adverse effect and a disadvantage to the use of hand sanitizers without proper consideration.

Harm to kids

Lots of hand sanitizers contain a high amount of ethanol or isopropyl alcohol, which you should keep out of reach of your kids, except there will be adult supervision. Children can require medical attention after using the sanitizers that contain a high level of alcohol.

Flammable items

The sanitizers contain a high level of alcohol content, which makes it flammable. Alcohol contains lots of combustible components. You should keep the product away from flame after purchase, such as a gas appliance or candle. You should not take a hand sanitizer to a barbecue grill or cooking space.

Tips for Using Hand Sanitizer effectively.

Firstly, apply the sanitizer to one of your hands.

Secondly, carefully rub your hands or palm jointly and ensure that you have covered every surface of your hands, including the back of your palm and all your fingers outside in.

However, Continue the process of rubbing it for at least for 30 to 60 seconds, pending your hands get dry. It can take almost 60 seconds or more, for hand sanitizer to eliminate or most germs.

Fourthly, all organic or germs matter is out from your hands, all visible bacteria.

What germs can hand sanitizer kill?

By CDC TRUSTED, hand sanitizers will not get bright or rid of potentially unsafe chemicals. It is also not valid at eliminating the following terms:

Norovirus

cryptosporidium (one of the germs that cause cryptosporidiosis)

clostridium difficile (also known or called as C. diff)

Sometimes, a hand sanitizer may not function well if your hands are dirty or greasy, oily, slippery. This may occur after eating food, doing daily or regular yard work, garden clearing, or playing a sport or games.

However, if your hands look dirty, oily or slimy, opt or ask for handwashing rather than a hand sanitizer.

Chapter 9: Are Hand Sanitizers Safe to Use?

Another thing that worries people is whether or not these products are actually safe to use, considering the chemicals used in production. Now, the CDC and the World Health Organization promote the use of hand sanitizers based on alcohol instead of the alcohol-free versions, since the free versions include more of these chemicals and some research suggested that some compound, like triclosan, interfere with our endocrine system, other than presenting an environmental concern. There is also the fact that excessive use of antimicrobial compounds stimulates the microbes to develop resistance to the formula, something that is becoming concerning in the modern world and that we need to promote the least possible.

At the same time, are alcohol-based products free from criticisms? Well, alcohol is flammable, and can be poisonous if ingested, that posed some safety concerns mainly in regard to children, or by people that seek to abuse of alcohol, however, with proper safety precautions, correct storage, and the proper education, these lines of products are considered to be much safer and to pose less of a risk than alcohol-free versions.

Be careful though, excessive use of alcohol-based products will deprive our skin of natural oils and in some cases, cause cracks, which are entry points for bacteria. So, keep your hands clean, but be moderate about it.

Safety measures of Homemade Hand Sanitizers

You should take a lot of care when using/handling essential oil. Essential oils are very concentrated extracts from plants. If not properly mixed can irritate your skin when it gets into contact with it. Essential oil should be used, especially with kids when diluted.

Make sure to always add an emulsifier to any essential oil you intend to use on your skin. Also, when an emulsifier is added to the essential oil, it becomes safe to be used on clothes thereby eliminating any fear of stain.

Disinfect the spoon, bowl, container and funnel properly before use with boiling water, as boiled water is sufficient enough to kill, protozoa, viruses and pathogenic bacteria.

Remember that the hand sanitizer should not replace washing hands. It can dry and as well cause some injury to the skin of your hands so you should only use it when only its needed.

Make sure it does not go into your eyes. In case it gets into your eyes, immediately wash it out and also seek medical attentions as soon as possible.

Things You Didn't Know About Sanitizers

Dosage and Ingredients Both Matter

Speaking of the products used in hand sanitizers, perhaps the only thing that counts is what is in your favorite formula. Of course, as stated, you want at least 60 per cent alcohol to get a sanitizer. The correct dosage is around a dollop of a quarter to a half-dollar scale. This would serve to cover the whole hands full. Having a little bit under the nails is always good.

Hand Sanitizers are Safe for Babies

Babies have very fragile and sensitive hands, but it does not mean they will not be able to profit from the hand sanitizers. Although the risk of alcohol consumption is relatively high, babies and even small children under the age of 6 barely show any significant consequences from exposure. Also, you do not want to overdo it of course. Make sure you are utilizing minimal doses of hand sanitizer, and your kids will be safe.

Hand Sanitizers Help to Protect Against Flu

Hand sanitizers provide decent, but not absolute, safety since the flu virus is airborne. While using a hand sanitizer to remove germs and viruses will be a part of your everyday health-conscious practice, make sure it is not the only thing you are doing. Germs are everywhere; security needs to be multifaceted and cover on the body not just the hands but also the neck and other places too.

Chapter 10: For Hand Disinfection

2/3 Cup 99% Isopropyl Alcohol to Rub In 1/3 Cup Aloe or Witch Hazel Gel

This recipe is very simple. Nothing special. Isopropyl alcohol, which helps kill germs and Aloe Vera or witch hazel to prevent the alcohol from evaporating too quickly before it evaporates completely after being rubbed into the skin.

Other recipes include fragrance oils and vitamin E that make the skin soft. None of these ingredients are required, but when mixed, the proposed combinations make an effective and convenient hand sanitizer. When purchasing oils, use essential oils as they are intended for use on the skin and no other fragrance oils that are intended for use in oil heaters and oil diffusers.

Here is a list of some essential oils and what is known to help mood control if you know this before disinfecting your hands.

Citrus - You can help improve your mood and feel more alert and energetic.

Mint - It can help calm the mood and increase energy.

Lavender - Can help you relax.

Rose Oil - It can help you relax and improve your mood.

Bergamot (sometimes called Lemon Leech) - It can help you improve your mood and relieve anxiety.

Vetiver (like lemongrass) - Can help increase energy and relieve anxiety.

Clary (sometimes called Sage) - It can help improve mood and promote a sense of peace.

Ylang-ylang - It can help mood, and in some it can be an aphrodisiac.

Incense - can help you feel grounded, promote relaxation and help depression.

Jasmine - It can help you lift your mood and depression.

Rosemary – perhaps help for improvement of concentration, fatigues, depression

Nice hand disinfectant

10 drops of peppermint oil 10 drops of vitamin E oil.

2/3 cup isopropyl alcohol 1/3 cup aloe vera gel

Mint - It can help calm the mood and increase energy.

A BEAUTIFUL LAVENDER DISINFECTANT

10 drops of lavender oil 5 drops of tea tree oil

5 drops of vitamin E oil 2/3 cup of isopropyl alcohol

1/3 cup aloe vera gel

Lavender - Can help you relax.

Disinfect the jasmine hand

10 drops of jasmine oil 5 drops of vitamin E oil.

2/3 cup isopropyl alcohol 1/3 cup aloe vera gel

Jasmine - It can help you lift your mood and depression.

Hand disinfection

10 drops of nutmeg oil 5 drops of vitamin E oil

2/3 cup isopropyl alcohol 1/3 cup aloe vera gel

Grass - It can help you improve your mood and promote calm feelings.

WHO RECOMMENDS MANUAL REGULATION?

1 cup of isopropyl alcohol

1 tablespoon of 3 percent hydrogen peroxide 1 tablespoon of 98% glycerin

¼ cup of distilled water

* METRO

The mixing instructions are similar to the recipes above, and use a glass, ceramic, or alcohol-resistant bowl to mix the ingredients.

DIY hand disinfectant wipes

If you want to disinfect your hands, but are looking for an alternative to conventional disinfectants, you can easily make your own disinfectant wipes. You will need things.

Fragrant baby wipes (Vitamin E has already been added to most baby wipes, making it an additional bonus for the skin.)

Depending on where you get the wipes, the number of wipes in the pack will vary, but this solution will hold about 30 wipes.

1/2 cup isopropyl alcohol

Ziploc bags (or if you have a cloth in a hard-plastic container, you can use it instead)

If you have handkerchiefs, just pour alcohol on the handkerchiefs and shake to cover them. Because the wipes are pre-wetted, it takes some time for the alcohol to become fully saturated, but this happens over time.

DIY surface disinfectant wipes

Why should you clean your hands when everything you touch is dirty and infected with germs? Creating tissues is easy and because people are becoming healthier and working The need to disinfect wipes will surely remain disease-free and will surely exceed the range on offer. Here is a quick recipe to make as many disinfectant wipes as you want.

1/2 cup of water

3/4 cup of isopropyl alcohol

1 teaspoon of anti-wrinkle dishwashing liquid 10 drops of lemon or citrus oil 2 tablespoons of ammonia (optional)

10-12 cloths or rags (You can use it to mount a used container. In addition, thicker rags absorb more fluid, so you may need fewer rags or washcloths. You can buy a rag from Walmart or a similar store for a few dollars.

A plastic container with a lid that can be hermetically sealed.

Put all the rags in the container and pour all the ingredients on the rags.

Attach the lid and shake vigorously to fully saturate it.

These wipes are reusable. Therefore, use them as usual for disposable wipes. When you are done, just throw them in the laundry.

If you prefer disposable towels, this recipe is enough to cover and saturate a standard roll of paper towels.

Some questions people ask

How long does the disinfectant expire?

Hand disinfection does not really take place. The date on the bottle is likely to end because hand disinfectants have been regulated by the FDA and certain items, including the expiration date, will need to be added to the packaging. The expiry date is the last date that the product contains the ingredient in the amount specified on the label. Either the manufacturer has proven to what extent the product complies with the label declaration, or it has simply set a random date to determine that the expiry date is unknown to consumers.

According to its protection data, alcohol is a stable chemical substance.

Sigma Aldrich Chemicals distribution sheet. This means that when the alcohol is stored in a container at room temperature, it remains in the same concentration for a very long time. However, alcohol evaporates easily because its boiling point is relatively low. Sometimes opening and closing the bottle can release different alcohols and the alcohol concentration during hand disinfection can decrease. However, if you can keep the bottle closed and at room temperature, you are likely to have an effective product for as long as you need it. Is hand disinfectant toxic to the skin?

Alcohols are considered safe as an antiseptic and do not affect the skin.

However, according to the database of hazardous substances, continuous use can lead to irritation or slight dryness. Many studies have shown that the constant use of hand disinfectants is less disruptive than the continuous washing of hands with soap. Damaged skin is more prone to irritation than alcohol. And to be honest, would you rather have a mild skin irritation or share and infect the disease?

You can choose ...

How to prevent the spread of coronavirus in households and shared apartments

A patient confirmed by COVID-19 in a symptomatic laboratory.

About

The patient to be examined.

Caregivers, close partners and household members outside of the medical community can have close contact with a confirmed person COVID-19 or an investigator. Close contacts should monitor their health or call a doctor if they experience symptoms similar to COVID-19, such as: fever to cough

Dyspnea

Ingredients for cleaning the face and how to use it

The ingredients for the manufacture of washcloths are widely used in all major brands, especially in drugstores.

Some ingredients are not expensive and can be obtained from petrochemicals. Another thing about wet wipes is that most people do not because of the nature of the product, which is very weak against mold and mildew, which means that you need to use strong and effective preservatives to make it work.

Ingredients and uses

pins

Propylene glycol

Parabens

A synthetic fragrance

Sticks: Sticks are glycols that help the formula penetrate, while carcinogenic contaminants are the main problem. When applied to damaged skin, they can cause pain and total toxicity.

2.Propylene Glycol: This ingredient is mainly found in many unnatural wet wipes and various other cosmetic products because it helps the ingredients through the skin.

3.Parabens: As mentioned above, wet wipes need intensive maintenance, so the presence of parabens in wet wipe preparations should be outdated. So, my opinion on this is better so that you are safe. I am not sorry.

Application

If you do not find disinfectant in the shops next door, you can do the same. You only need a few ingredients such as essential oil or lemon juice, alcohol and aloe vera gel. Hand disinfection is very helpful in preventing germs from spreading when soap and water are not available. Alcohol-based hand disinfectants can be very helpful in ensuring safety and slowing the spread of the new corona virus. Although hand disinfectants can be an effective way of removing germs, health care providers still recommend washing your hands to keep your hands free from diseases that cause viruses and many other germs. Be sure!

Conclusion

Health is wealth, you hear people say; at this time, no one really cares about wealth. All they care about is being healthy. In this book, we have provided you with details that will help you stay healthy at all times. That is why we have spent more time on helping you with information that will help you stay protected. You have been informed on how to wash your hands effectively, which will protect you from contracting the virus that has been killing thousands of people worldwide.

We have also considered how to make your hand sanitizer from home. The use of sanitizer is one of the best ways to keep yourself protected from getting infected with any virus whatsoever.

The truth is getting a sanitizer from stores at this time is hard. So, you should pay attention to preparing your own from home. We have delivered the essential ingredients you need to make your homemade hand sanitizer

The trick to keeping any rapid spreading viruses and infections away is by being conscious of your hygiene. Stocking up on homemade hand sanitizer is one way to do this and it is important to extend this habit to your children, or direct family members.

The areas we overlook and are often the exact ways we contract bugs and by not keeping other, regularly used items clean. Items such as mobile phones, and money (plastic and paper) which we are rarely without.

Keeping your bathroom, and kitchen space clean are other ways to avoid viruses. Spraying any surface with an antibacterial or antimicrobial cleaning product will ensure that you kill any lurking germs.

The biggest barrier against disease is by becoming a bit stricter with your hygiene habits. Wash your hands, sanitize and stay indoors when ill.

There you have it, make sure you follow the instructions. The alcohol content for making the sanitizers should be at least 70%.

Ensure that you shake the bottle before squeezing out the sanitizer.

All surfaces around your house and office should be regularly cleaned with sanitizer.

Consider making some for your friends and family members too.

Stay safe and practice good personal hygiene. Do not forget to teach your children to keep good hygiene. Teach them to wash their hand before touching their own bodies, such as eyes and mouth. The use of hand sanitizers for hand washing helps to reduce the spread of bacteria and microorganisms in various manners.

The regular hand washing we do by making use of our antiseptic soap just helps to remove the bacteria off our hands.

The hand sanitizer, on the other hand, does things differently. It does not wash the bacteria off your hands, but it eradicates the bacteria chemically, thereby intensely reducing the level of microbes on your hand.

It is almost like making use of germicides to disinfect the surroundings and surfaces to keep them germ-free.

The importance of hand washing is based on the soap application and the timeframe for washing. Imagine washing your hands without making use of soap; it is wrong because it is not a practical approach.

Finally, if you found this book useful in any way, a review on Amazon is always appreciated!

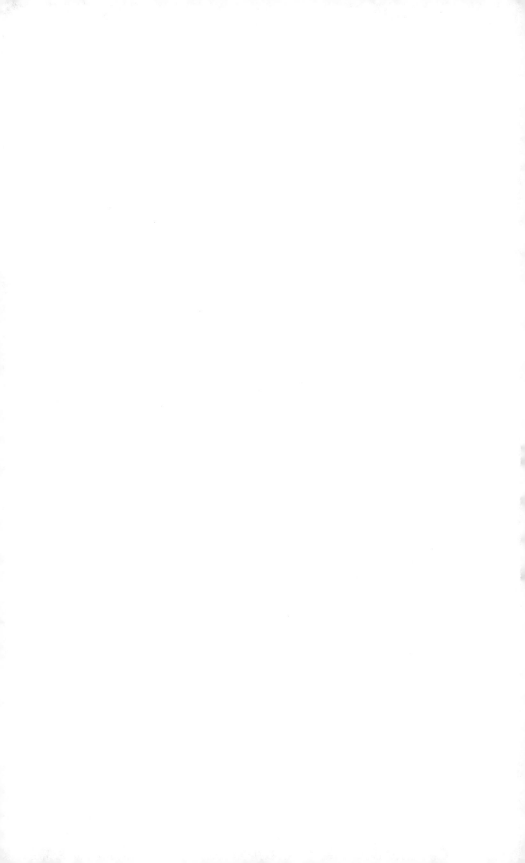